Strategies to Treat Psoriasis and Psoriatic Arthritis

Strategies to Treat Psoriasis and Psoriatic Arthritis

Everything You Wish Your Doctor Had Told You

Dr. Diana Hurwitz and Dr. Jill Weintraub

Waterside Productions

First Printing, 2022

ISBN-13: 978-1-958848-17-3 print edition
ISBN-13: 978-1-958848-18-0 e-book edition

Waterside Productions
2055 Oxford Ave
Cardiff, CA 92007
www.waterside.com

Dedication

We dedicate this book to our patients who have entrusted us with their care, and inspire us to incorporate mind, body, and spirit into the art of medicine. Thank you for allowing us to be a part of your lives.

Contents

Introduction ix
Meet the Authors xi
Let's Start at the Beginning: What is the Psoriasis/ Psoriatic Arthritis Disease Spectrum? xiii

Part 1: Co-Associated Disorders of Psoriasis and Psoriatic Arthritis: Cardiac Disease and Mental Health 1
Part 2: Dietary and lifestyle choices we recommend to our patients with psoriasis and psoriatic arthritis 3
Part 3: Recipes: Recipes that can help control psoriasis and psoriatic arthritis 25

INTRODUCTION

A dermatologist and a rheumatologist combine their clinical and personal experiences with evidence based medicine to help you take control over your psoriasis and psoriatic arthritis.

Dr. Diana Hurwitz, a board-certified Dermatologist, and Dr. Jill Weintraub Landis, a double board-certified Integrative Rheumatologist, share their 40+ years of combined clinical experience in treating psoriasis and psoriatic arthritis to help you control your symptoms, understand your triggers and reduce your risk of developing long term complications.

Why did we start this project? We began collaborating on mutual patients who had psoriasis and psoriatic arthritis over a decade ago. We found that taking a collaborative approach was a powerful tool in giving our mutual patients the benefit of our combined experience. (We can also relate personally: Diana has Celiac disease and Jill's mother has suffered with psoriatic arthritis for many years.)

In our many discussions, we discovered that our medications worked much better in people who were actively involved in maintaining their overall health through lifestyle and dietary choices. We also noticed that many patients did not have the tools they needed to make those informed choices. Because of this, we researched which dietary and lifestyle choices were the most pertinent for people with the psoriasis-psoriatic disease spectrum, and gave them to our patients. What we found is that those who had this actionable information were better able to understand their disease process, and what triggers it. We also noticed that armed with this information, and the knowledge that they could get better, people with psoriasis and psoriatic arthritis responded better to their medications and had fewer complications.

This is an exciting time for psoriasis and psoriatic arthritis as major advances are being made for new systemic treatments. However, these medications work much better as part of a combined approach, including lifestyle and dietary management. The details provided in this ebook are backed by evidence, research, and our clinical acumen and will empower you to get the most out of your doctor visits, identify what triggers your symptoms, and integrate holistic healing methods into your life. We wrote this book to give you the tools to start these conversations with your doctors and actively participate in your health. It's what we wanted for our patients, ourselves, and our families. Now we're giving it to you.

Meet the Authors

Meet Dr. Diana Hurwitz

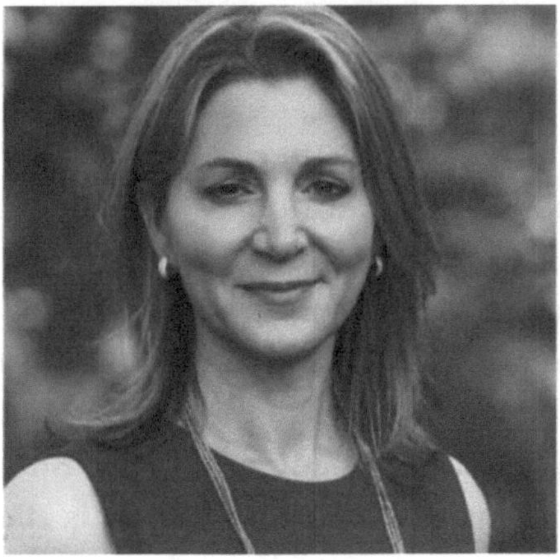

Dr. Diana Hurwitz is a board certified Dermatologist. She completed her undergraduate education at Harvard College with honors. She continued on to Mount Sinai School of Medicine after taking a year to work on psychopharmacology at Massachusetts General Hospital. She finished her internal medicine residency at Yale New Haven Hospital and completed her dermatology residency at the University of Miami. She was the chief of dermatology at a large multi-specialty group for over ten years and has been named one of New York's best doctors multiple times. Dr Hurwitz has integrated complementary medicine into her practice and co-founded Kitchen-Prescription, a cooking and wellness blog, to share her passion and expertise on food as medicine.

Meet Dr. Jill Weintraub

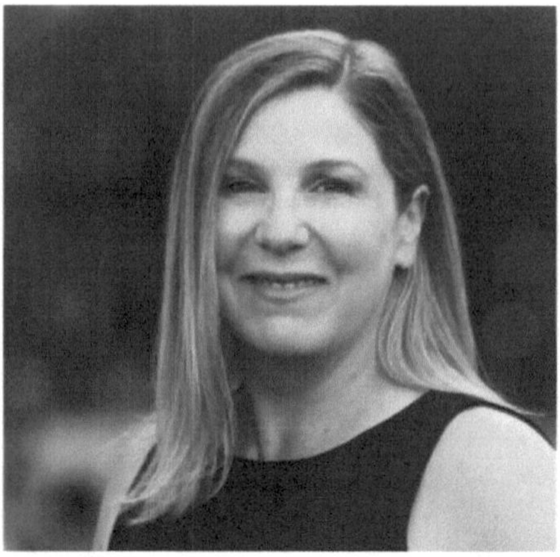

Dr. Jill Weintraub Landis is a double board-certified Integrative Rheumatologist. She completed her undergraduate training at the University of Michigan, and continued on to the Albert Einstein College of Medicine, where she graduated with honors. She finished her Internal Medicine Residency at The Mount Sinai Medical Center and completed her Rheumatology subspecialty training at The Hospital for Joint Disease at NYU. She is the Andrew Lowell fellowship recipient for the study of Integrative Medicine with Dr. Andrew Weil. She was the Chief of Rheumatology at a large multispecialty group for over 10 years, and named one of New York's best doctors. Dr. Weintraub is an active member of the American College of Rheumatology, and the primary investigator for several studies on the use of complementary therapies in autoimmune diseases. She is also a trained chef and the founder of Integrative Rheumatology Consultants at http://www.jillweintraubmd.com, and is the co-creator of Kitchen-Prescription, a cooking and wellness blog.

Let's Start at the Beginning What is the Psoriasis/Psoriatic Arthritis Disease Spectrum?

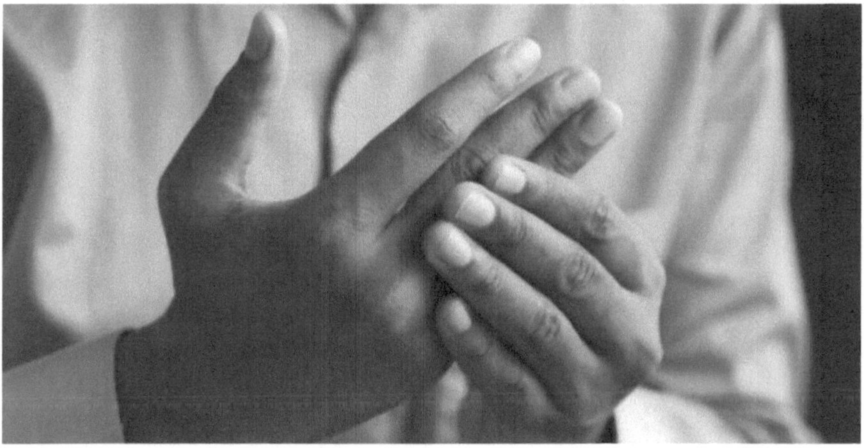

Psoriasis and Psoriatic Arthritis are inflammatory disorders that target not only the skin and joint but can also affect the spine, eyes, and gastrointestinal (GI) tract. They are caused by a combination of genetic, environmental, hormonal, and dietary factors. Untreated chronic inflammation over time can lead to obesity, heart disease, strokes, diabetes, and significant mental health issues. In other words, psoriasis/psoriatic arthritis is a syndrome that goes way beyond skin and joints. We think about it as a whole body disorder that affects many organs and can lead to significant disability, if left untreated.

Although psoriasis affects up to 3.2% of the U.S. population, patients are frequently undiagnosed, under treated, or untreated altogether, with many being unaware that they have psoriatic arthritis in addition to skin involvement. Over 30% of people with psoriasis have co-associated tendonitis and inflammatory arthritis, which can affect both small and large joints, as well as the spine. Psoriasis can also co-exist with inflammatory bowel disease (IBD), sometimes subclinical, or too mild to be diagnosed, and uveitis, or inflammatory eye disease.

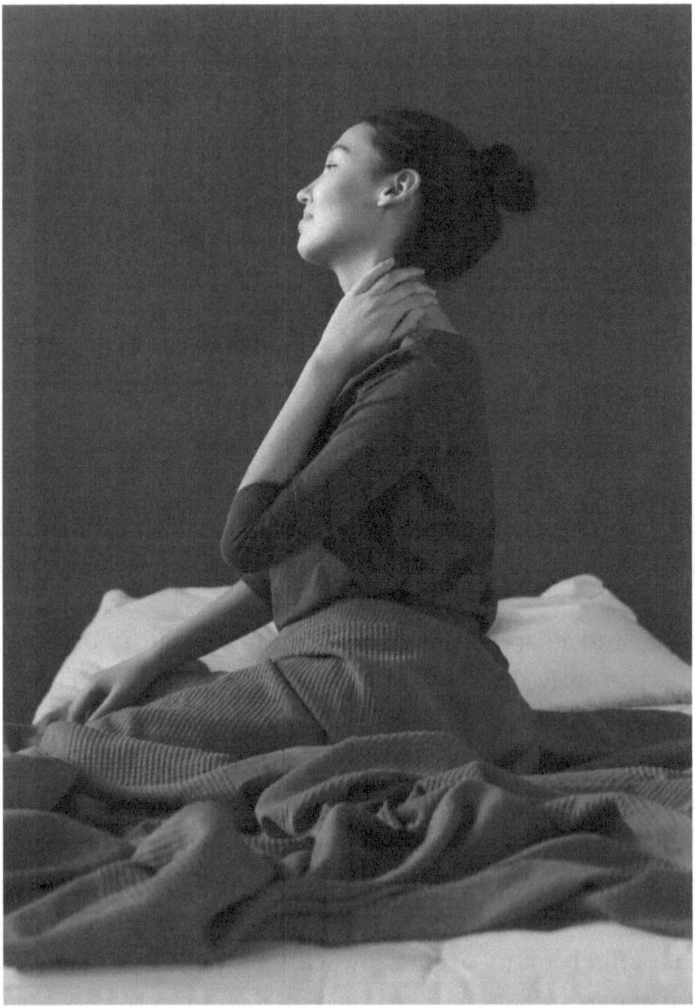

Patient vignette: DK is a 45 year old construction worker with a ten year history of skin psoriasis. He has suffered with lower back pain for over ten years, has trouble getting out of bed in the morning, feels stiff and sore for a few hours and notices that the pain lessened by the afternoon. He always chalked it up to a work-related injury. "I've had psoriasis for over ten years and never knew that my back pain was related. It wasn't until I was referred to a rheumatologist that I realized I also had psoriatic arthritis." DK

Impacted individuals typically first experience symptoms on their skin or joints, but this chronic disease can negatively impact several other areas of a person's health and overall quality of life as well.

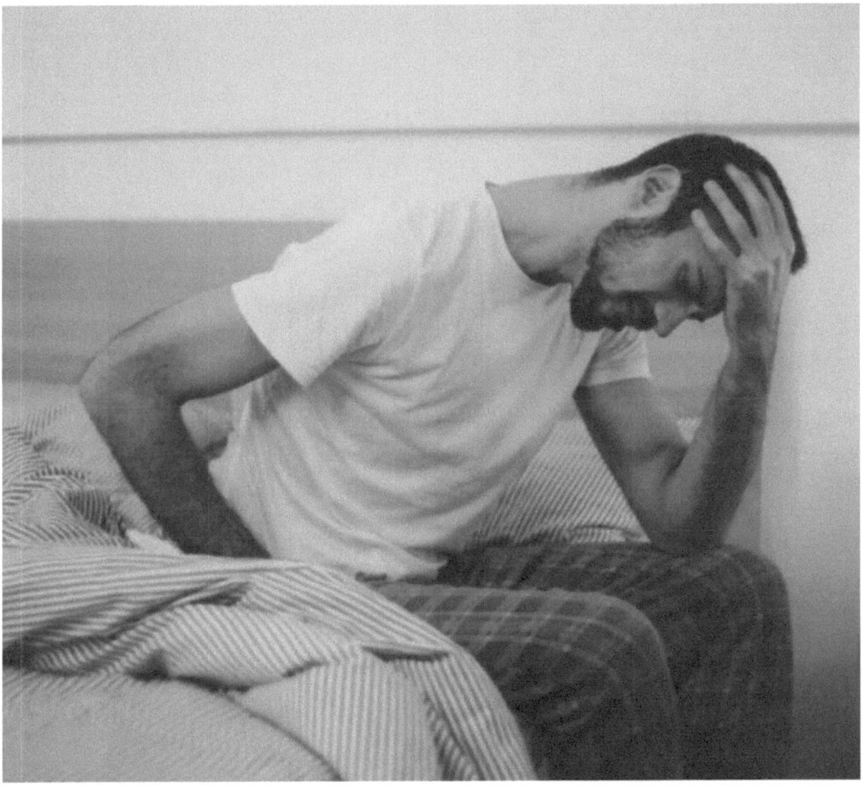

Part 1: Co-Associated Disorders of Psoriasis and Psoriatic Arthritis: Cardiac Disease and Mental Health

There is a growing awareness of the connection between psoriasis/psoriatic arthritis and cardiovascular disease. This is likely due to the body's overactive inflammatory response which can lead to hardening of the arteries. The American Heart Association and American College of Cardiology have recently identified chronic inflammatory diseases such as psoriasis as a major risk factor for contracting heart disease.

How do psoriasis and psoriatic arthritis impact mental health?

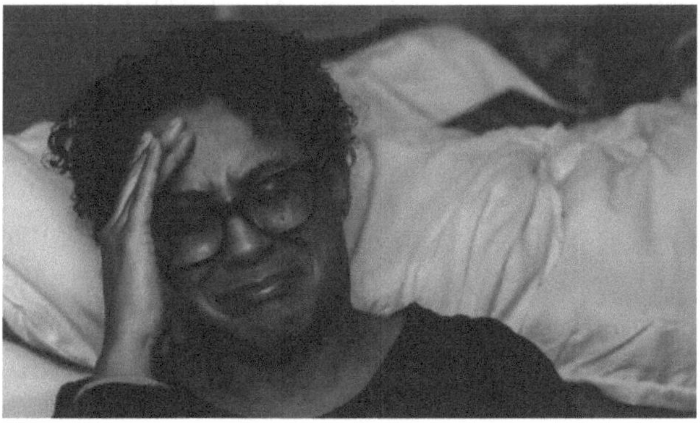

Psoriasis affects the personal, social, and sexual lives of the patients resulting in significant psychological strain. Social stigmatization and low self-esteem play a real role in causing depression in people with psoriasis. Many are ashamed of their disease, which contributes to social isolation, anxiety, and helplessness. In fact, psoriatics are 1.5x more likely to be depressed. Depression may manifest as mood changes, increasing pain, or more fatigue. Managing the psychosocial part of this illness, along with the physical aspects, leads to better treatment outcomes.

Patient vignette: Lily is a 35 year old single social worker with psoriasis. "I was so ashamed of my skin condition especially after a friend asked me whether my skin rash was contagious. I reassured her it was not, but it magnified my fears of exposing my skin in public. I was also afraid to date because I didn't want to show my skin, and be judged by my appearance. I realized these fears contributed to my social isolation and my depression. When I finally got help for both my skin and my depression, my life turned around." L

Those who have Psoriasis and Psoriatic Arthritis can often suffer from the following health conditions:

- Cardio metabolic syndrome
- Fatty liver
- Heart disease
- Diabetes
- High cholesterol levels (hyperlipidemia)
- Obesity
- Fatigue
- Colitis
- Eye Inflammation/ Uveitis
- Gout
- Hashimoto's Disease
- Celiac Disease
- SLE (Systemic Lupus Erythematosus)
- Other autoimmune disorders
- Metabolic Syndrome (High blood pressure, insulin resistance, increased lipids in the blood

Part 2:
Dietary and lifestyle choices we recommend to our patients with psoriasis and psoriatic arthritis

Now that we've defined psoriasis and psoriatic arthritis and explained how it impacts individuals, let's dive into how to support it by looking at foods and lifestyle choices that impact the disease. This is an action plan that includes the medications you may already take, as well as holistic treatment options. In our experience, this combination works best together.

Work closely with your doctor to see if a Systemic Therapy is right for you.

And, here is a list of potential issues related to psoriasis and psoriatic arthritis to discuss with your doctor during your office visit:

- **Screen for drugs that worsen psoriasis** (these may include lithium, beta-blockers, antimalarials, interferon, and rapid tapers of systemic corticosteroids, among others).
- Screen for celiac disease and gluten sensitivity
- Check HLA b27 status (which is a blood test that looks for a protein found on white blood cells). If present, you will need annual screening for uveitis, or inflammation of the eye.
- Screen for depression

- Screen for hypertension
- Assess CRP
  (a marker of inflammation made by the liver)
- Evaluate for other cardiac risk factors
- Ask for help to quit smoking, if applicable
- Calculate BMI
- Test vitamin-D levels

Discuss techniques to avoid chronic joint pain, and the development of fibromyalgia, which is a separate musculoskeletal disorder caused by the brain's response to long standing bone and joint inflammation.

CONSIDER YOUR DIET

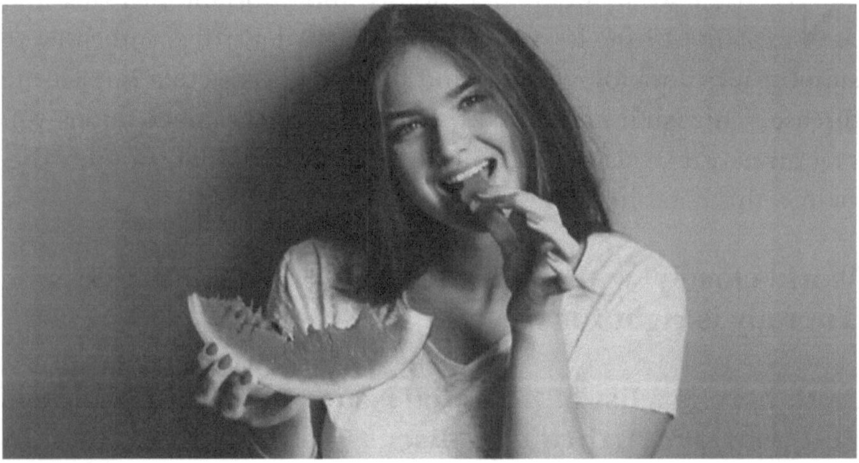

If you are experiencing psoriasis or psoriatic arthritis, think about avoiding or limiting the following:

- Sugar
- Alcohol
- Gluten
- Spicy foods
- Red Meat
- Dairy
- Fast food

Mediterranean Diet and Anti-Inflammatory Diet

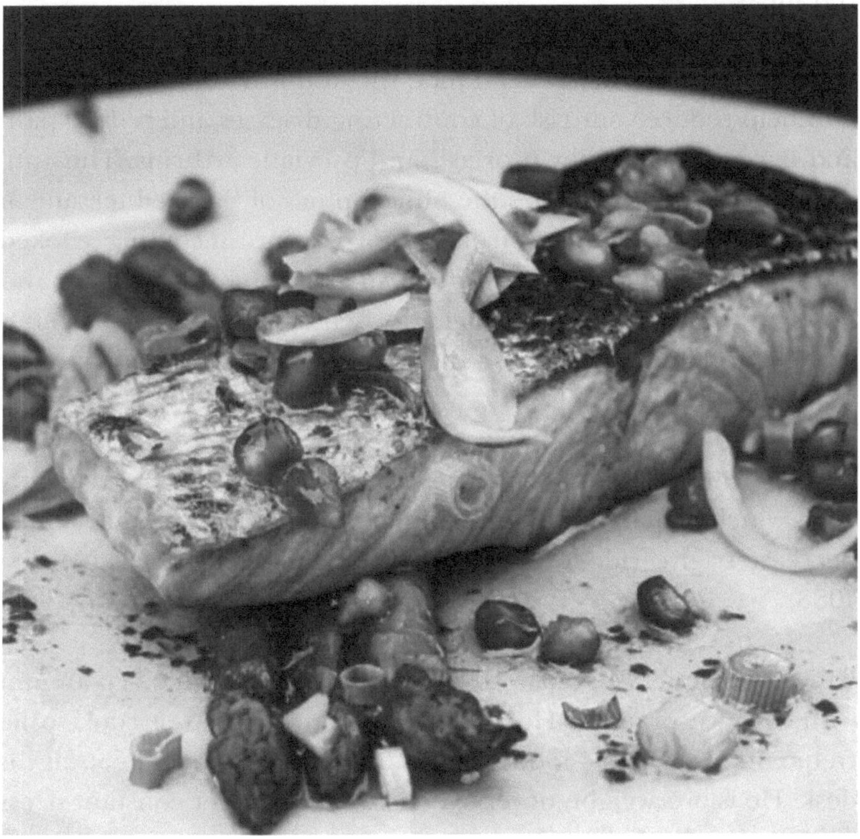

Prior to the introduction of fast food in Europe, individuals living in Greece and Italy had extremely healthy diets that made them far less susceptible to chronic diseases, when compared to Americans. Adopting a Mediterranean diet helps reduce inflammation and prevent the risk of heart attack, diabetes, and other illnesses.

The Mediterranean diet is a way of eating based on the traditional cuisine of countries bordering the Mediterranean Sea. The diet emphasizes daily consumption of vegetables, fruits, whole grains, and healthy fats with small portions of dairy and red meat.

Similar to the Mediterranean diet, the anti-inflammatory diet can also help reduce your risk of contracting diseases and reduce pain and flare ups caused by psoriasis and psoriatic arthritis. The anti-inflammatory diet includes the philosophies of the Mediterranean diet, as well as elements from Asian cuisine, including cooked mushrooms and whole soy products such as tofu. Chicken can also be included, but is best consumed when it is free range, vegetarian fed, and antibiotic free so that the microbiome is not adversely affected.

Salmon, sardines, tuna, and other fish are high in omega-3 fatty acids which help fight inflammation. Fish oil supplements also help decrease triglyceride levels and improve cholesterol levels (Ashley, 1988).

Patient vignette: Mike is a divorced 55 year old male accountant with his own practice. He works long hours, does not cook so he frequently eats at fast food restaurants or takes out and eats at his desk. He is overweight, never exercises and is under constant stress with tax deadlines looming.

When he is particularly stressed he craves burgers, fries and milkshakes. He has had psoriasis for over 20 years and suffered with chronic joint pain.

Finally, he was in so much pain he went to his doctor, was diagnosed with psoriatic arthritis in addition to his psoriasis diagnosis and put on a weight loss plan and an anti-inflammatory diet. "I feel so much more in control of my health and better in my own body since starting an anti-inflammatory diet. I also think that my medication works much better now." MB

Spices and Herbs

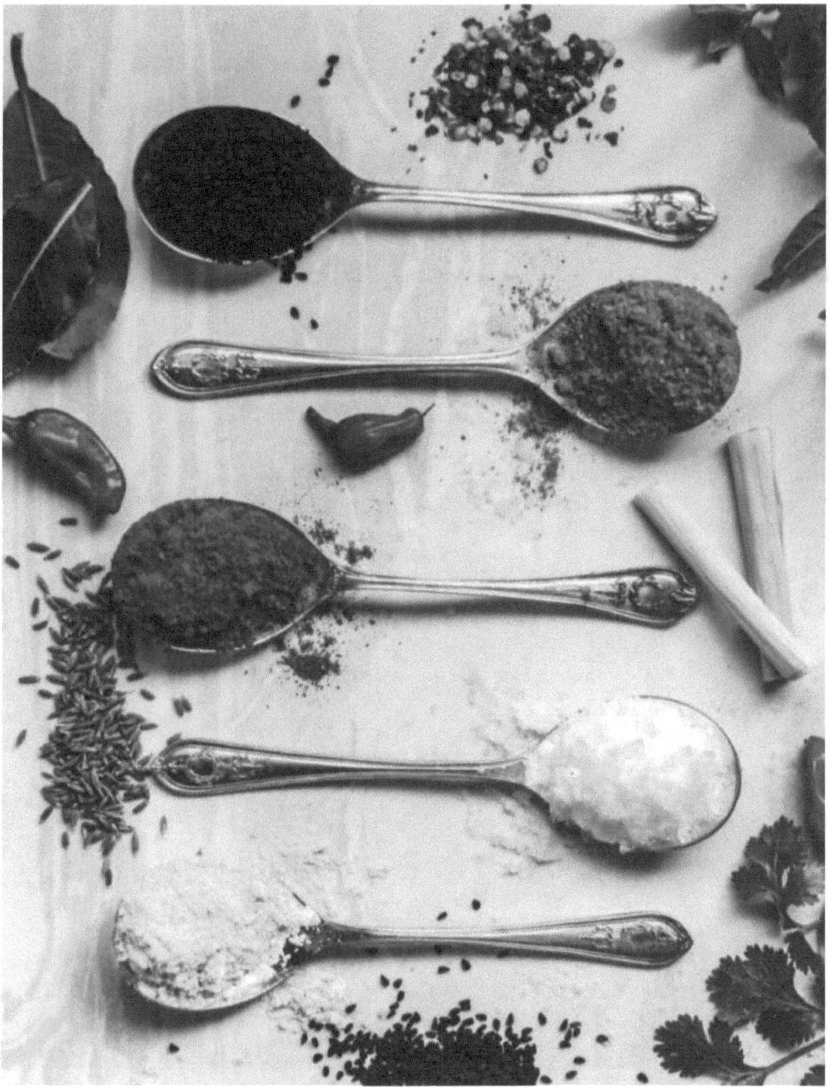

Natural herbs and spices such as thyme, sage, cumin, turmeric, and ginger help reduce inflammation and are a great addition to cooked meals. Turmeric contains an ingredient called curcumin that has strong anti-inflammatory properties.

Fruits & Vegetables

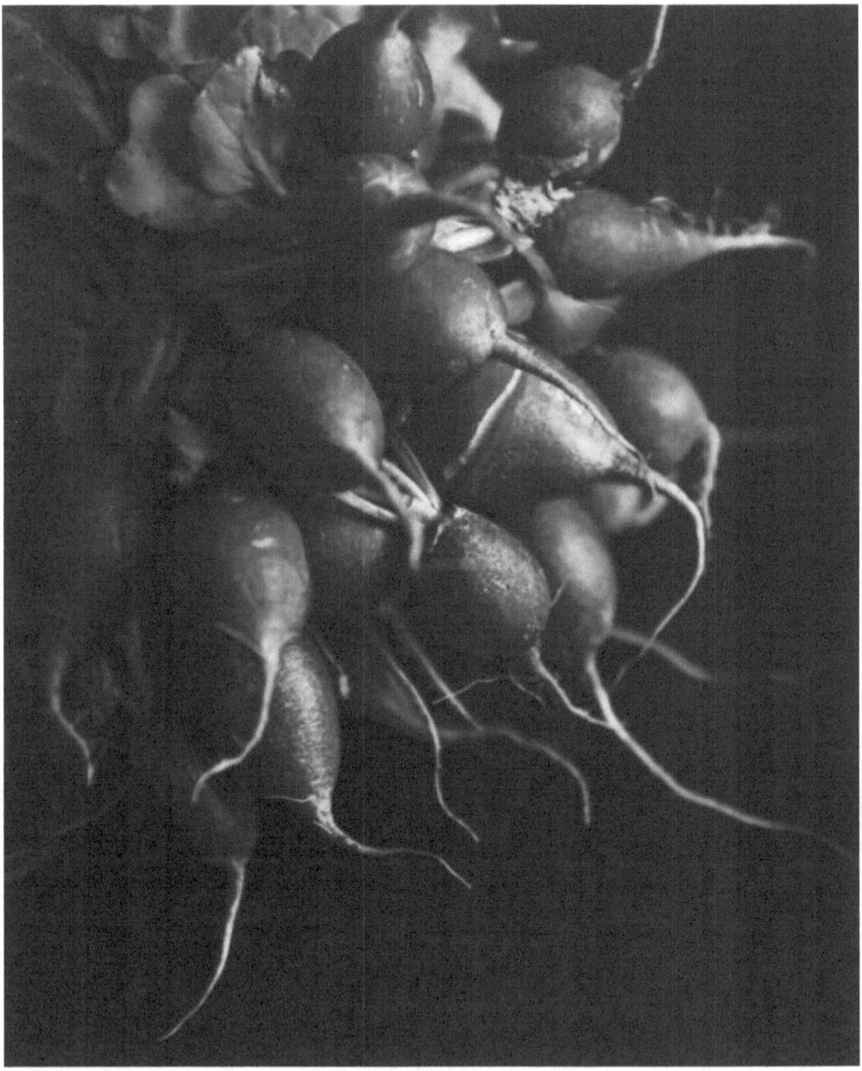

Fruits and vegetables are a great source of vitamins, minerals, phytonutrients, and fiber which help aid digestion, and maintain regular bowel movements.

They are the mainstay of an anti-inflammatory diet, and regular consumption can reduce chronic inflammation and lower long term cardiovascular and cancer risk.

SUPPORT YOUR MICROBIOME WITH PREBIOTICS & PROBIOTICS

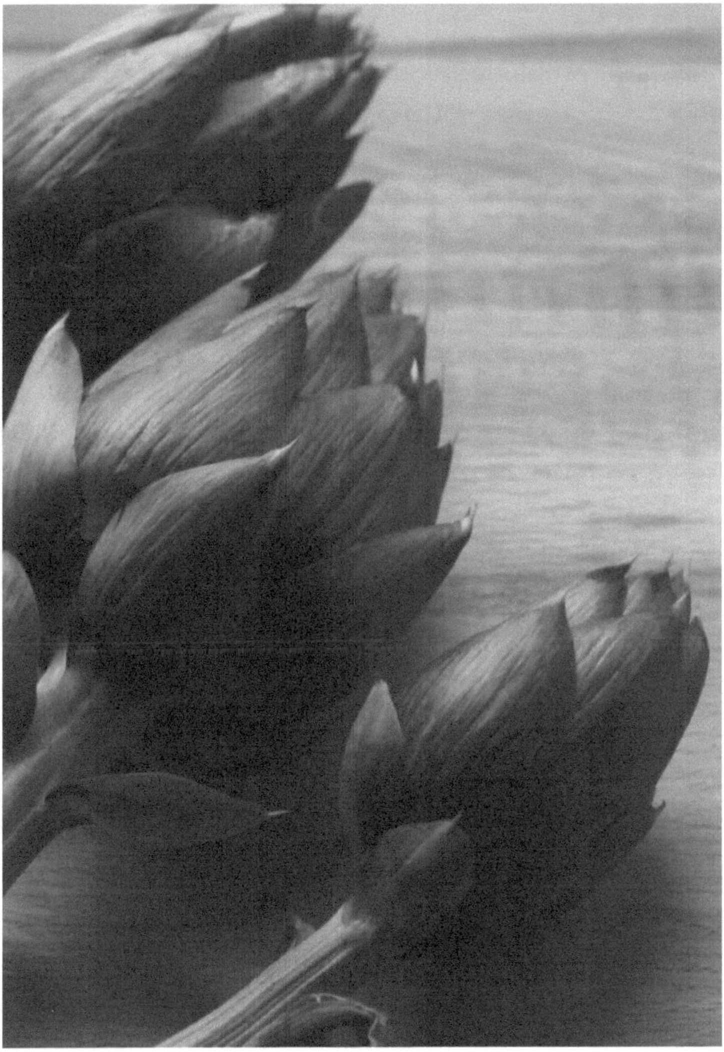

The microbiome is the collection of all the bacteria, fungi and viruses that normally live in our gut. These naturally occurring organisms help our body digest food, absorb nutrients, and neutralize toxins and unwanted bacteria.

This system is critical to the way our immune system functions, and keeps us healthy.

Prebiotic and probiotic foods support a healthy microbiome. Prebiotics are foods that nourish and provide structural support for the bacteria living in our gut. Prebiotic-rich foods include beans, leeks, onions, garlic, artichokes, bananas, flaxseeds, and other fiber-rich foods.

Probiotic foods contain more of the beneficial bacteria that already live naturally inside your gastrointestinal tract. Probiotic rich foods include fermented items such as yogurt, salt-preserved pickles, miso, kimchi, and kefir. Additionally, these items contain the metabolic by products of these good bacteria, including short-chain fatty acids. Short chain fatty acids provide nutritional support for the cells lining your GI tract, and may help maintain the integrity of the gut lining. This is important because maintaining that barrier prevents unwanted material from crossing the gut border, and interfacing with your body's immune system in a way that triggers unnecessary inflammation.

LOOK TO OTHER WHOLE MEDICINE SYSTEMS: TRADITIONAL CHINESE MEDICINE, AYURVEDA

Easy-to-Digest Foods

According to Traditional Chinese Medicine, good digestion is at the heart of maintaining health, and preventing inflammation.

Simplifying the diet to include whole grains, vegetables, and small amounts of animal protein is thought to be protective, as is eating cooked, wet foods that are easy to digest. Cold, raw, and spicy foods are thought to aggravate the intestinal tract, and should be avoided in the presence of psoriasis and psoriatic arthritis.

Ayurveda looks at health through the balance of Doshas, or three energies – Vata, Pitta, and Kapha – that circulate in the body and govern physiologic activity. Psoriasis and Psoriatic arthritis are inflammatory conditions characterized as an excess of Vata dosha. Vata dosha can be minimized through eating foods that emphasize the other doshas.

An Ayurvedic diet for psoriasis and psoriatic arthritis would inform patients to avoid acidic, sour foods, such as citrus fruits, and tomatoes, as well as dairy and meat products. Cooked rice, beans, and green vegetables prepared with unsaturated fats such as avocado oil are encouraged, as is the liberal drinking of warm water. Similar to Traditional Chinese Medicine, cold, raw, and spicy foods are to be avoided.

Pt vignette: Sara is a 45 year-old mother of two small children who has had trouble losing her postpartum baby weight. She struggles with feeding her family, and getting the nutrition she needs for herself as well. Her psoriatic arthritis has been more active since her last pregnancy. Her steady diet of raw salads and smoothies did not help joint pain or weight loss attempts, and often left her with indigestion. Switching to a primarily cooked-food diet including soups and stews aided her weight loss and made family meals easier. "Eating cooked foods instead of raw salads and smoothies has made my stomach feel so much better. I no longer feel hungry between meals and I'm much less bloated. My joint pain is lessened as well." SE.

KNOW WHAT YOU NEED TO AVOID

Fast Food

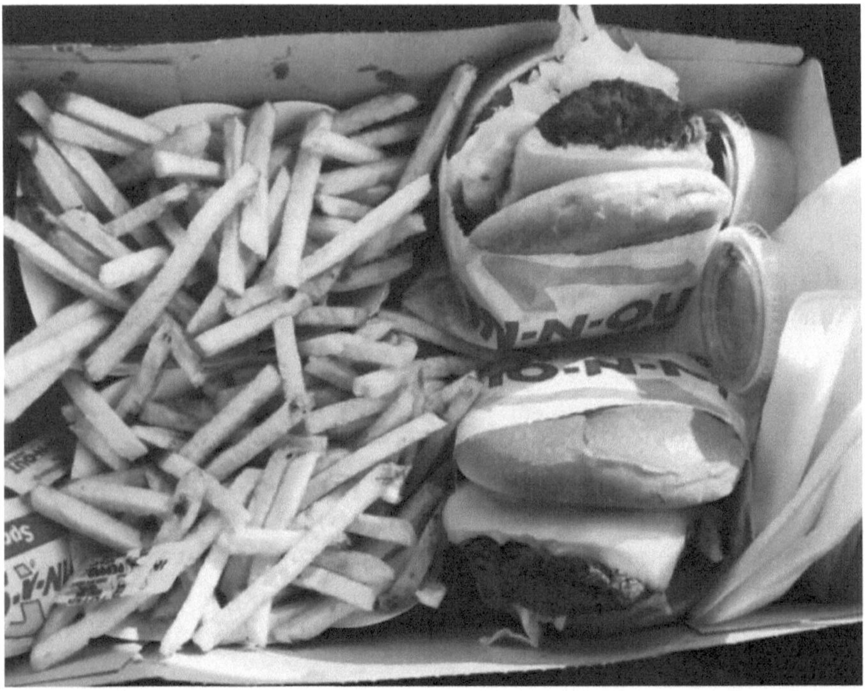

Fast food is cheap, easy and addictive and is amongst the most dangerous and toxic foods a person can eat. It has major repercussions on a person's health, even when consumed sparingly. With that being said, fast food is unfortunately an integral aspect of the Standard American Diet (SAD), with many consuming it several times per month or more. Although it is affordable, it is also loaded with sugar, salt, and fat which makes it highly addictive. This, in turn, has led to 42% of Americans being diagnosed with obesity, while more than 50% of Americans are currently overweight. Fast food, along with several of the other foods highlighted below, contributes to insulin resistance, high blood pressure, obesity, and inflammation, which can trigger psoriasis flare-ups.

SPECIFIC FOODS:

Oils

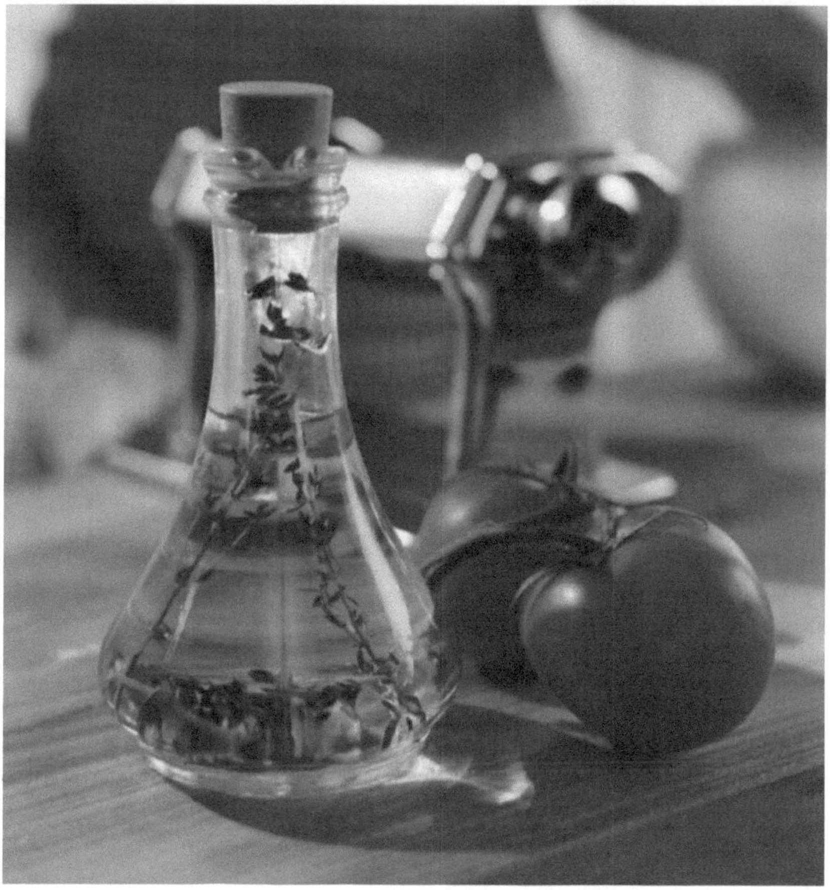

Cooking oils contain 3 types of fatty acids: omega-6, omega-3, and omega-9. Omega-6 fatty acids – which is found in corn, soybean, and canola oils – can be inflammatory, and are best avoided. Alternatively, omega-3 fatty acids – which are found in fatty fish like salmon, flax seeds, chia seeds, and walnuts, have anti-inflammatory properties, and should be included in any diet proposed for psoriasis and psoriatic arthritis.

Sugar

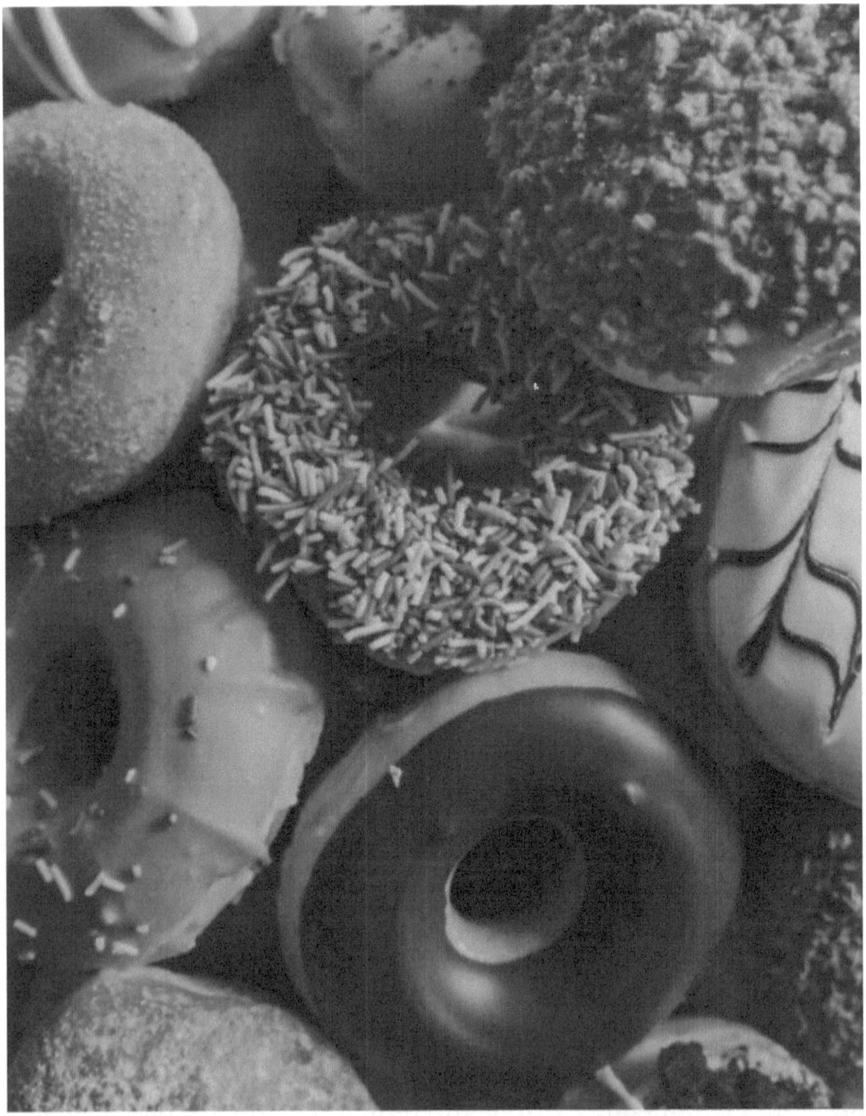

Just like fast food, sugar, including high fructose corn syrup, can drive inflammation leading to a flare of your psoriasis and psoriatic arthritis so try to reduce added sugar intake significantly. Better yet, eliminate it from your diet altogether – especially during flare-ups. We are not suggesting limiting natural sugars found in fruits however.

Gluten

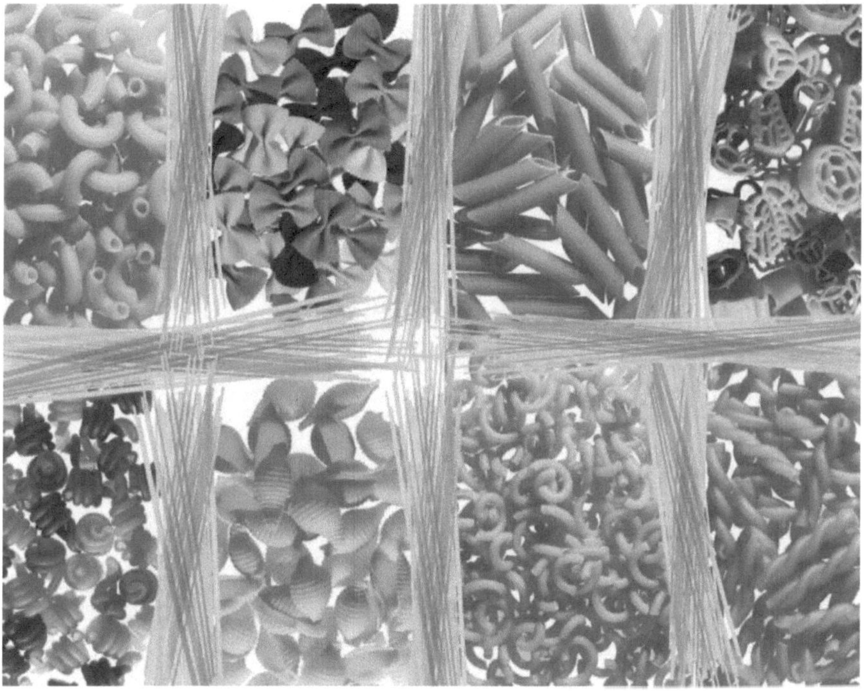

Individuals with psoriasis are at higher risk of contracting celiac disease. Even without celiac disease, some patients with psoriasis experience improvement on a gluten free diet (Bhatia, 2014), but this can vary person-to-person. This is a good discussion to have with your doctor. (Damasiewicz-Bodzek, 2008; Michaëlsson, 2003).

In our practice, we have found that some people respond very well to gluten free or low gluten diets, while it doesn't seem to matter at all for others.

Telling your doctor about family history of gluten sensitivity and gastrointestinal symptoms, diarrhea, and iron deficiency (anemia) is extremely helpful in identifying those who may be sensitive to gluten.

Patient vignette: Lynn is a 40 year old female lawyer with long standing psoriasis. She has a regular exercise routine, and is average weight but was frustrated by her lack of improvement in her skin clearance. She was very invested in her health, was in good general health but wanted her skin to be almost clear. She went on a gluten and dairy free diet, began taking a systemic drug, and went on an anti-inflammatory diet that involved eating more fish. After two visits, her skin was almost clear for the first time and she no longer complained of brain fog. She noticed her energy levels increased dramatically and she felt that her systemic medication was much more effective. LM

Nightshade Vegetables

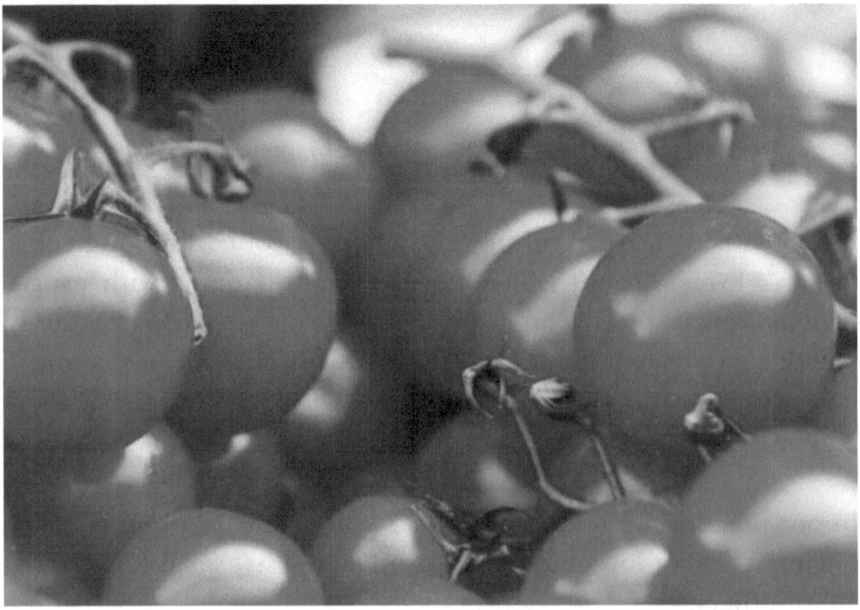

While it is important to consume fruits and vegetables to promote healing, there are certain vegetables – referred to as 'nightshades' – that may flare psoriasis and psoriatic arthritis symptoms. White potatoes, tomatoes, peppers, and eggplants are nightshade vegetables that contain solanine which may cause or exacerbate psoriasis and psoriatic arthritis in some people. It's important to pay attention to your symptoms when you eat these foods, to see if you need to eliminate them from your diet.

Red Meat & Dairy

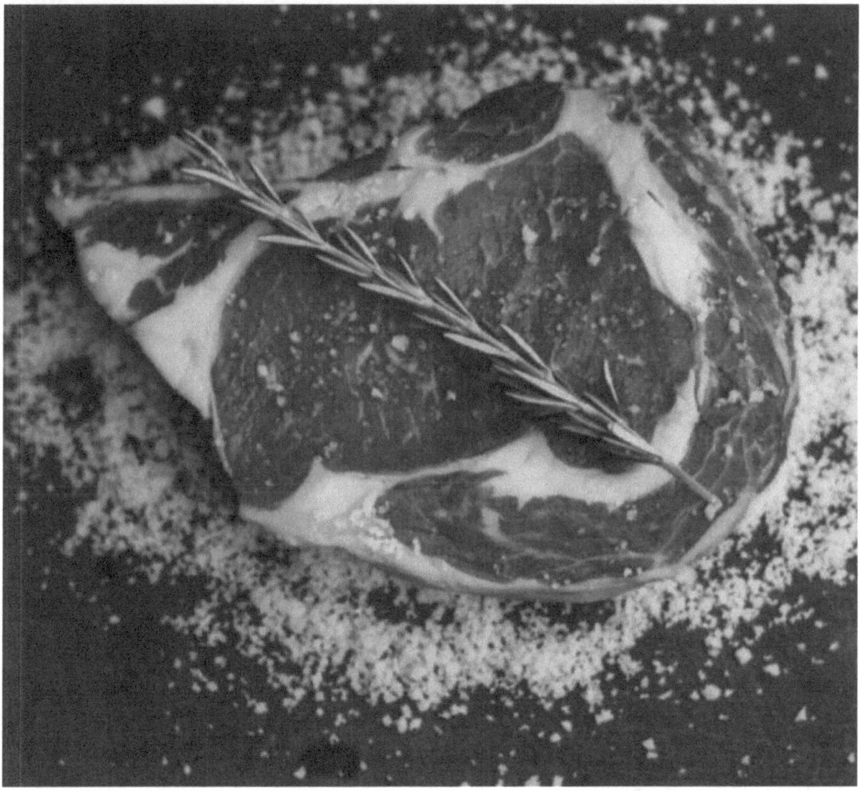

Avoid eating shrimp, beef, lamb, and other red meat, and consider limiting milk, eggs, cheese, and dairy. Yogurt, a fermented food, may be an exception to this. A diet that is rich in dairy and red meat leads to increased intake of saturated fats, which can exacerbate psoriasis and psoriatic arthritis.

A Word about Alcohol

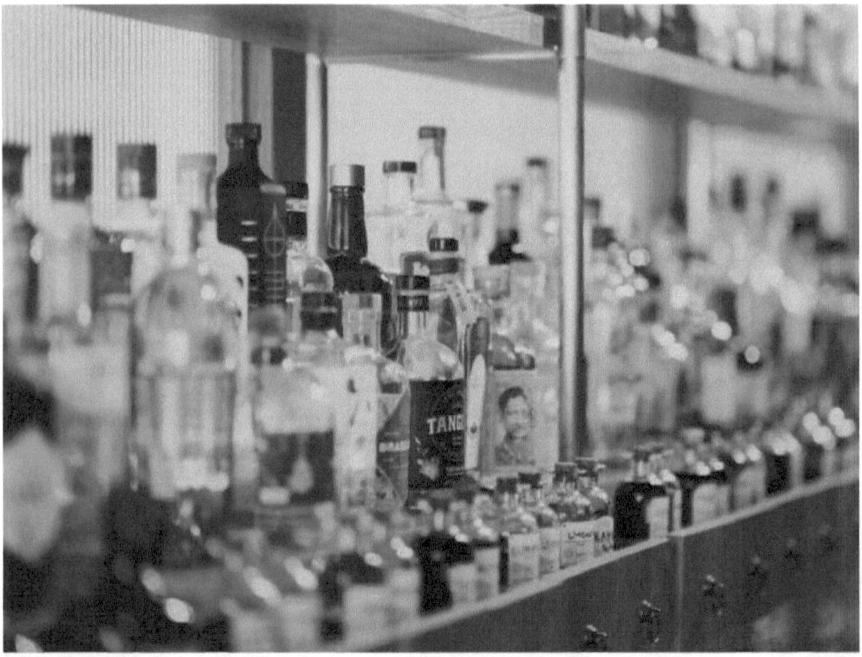

Alcohol is a very strong trigger for psoriasis. Fifteen case-controlled studies found a significant connection between alcohol consumption and the risk of developing psoriasis (Zhu, 2012). Other studies have found that alcohol may actually increase the body's resistance to treatment altogether. A study that followed 3,132 males and 2,555 females with psoriasis over 22 years found that those who consumed alcohol had a higher death rate than those who did not. (Poikolainen, 1999).

We recognize it can be difficult to cut out drinking altogether, especially while out to dinner or at social gatherings. During periods when flare ups are low, drinking occasionally and keeping consumption low shouldn't have a severe impact. However, during flare ups, it is best to cut out drinking entirely.

Medications to Avoid

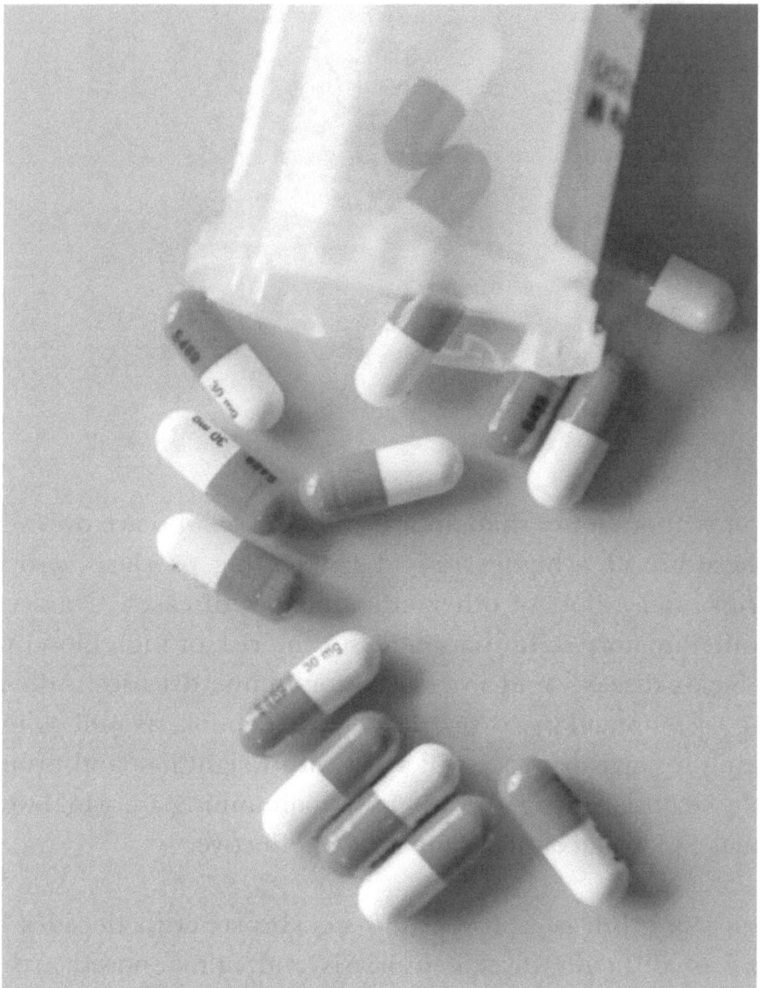

Beta blockers, lithium, NSAIDS, ACE inhibitors, antimalarials, and rapid steroid tapers can all cause psoriasis flare-ups. If you are taking any of these medications, speak with your doctor about how they may be contributing to your psoriasis symptoms.

Weight Loss

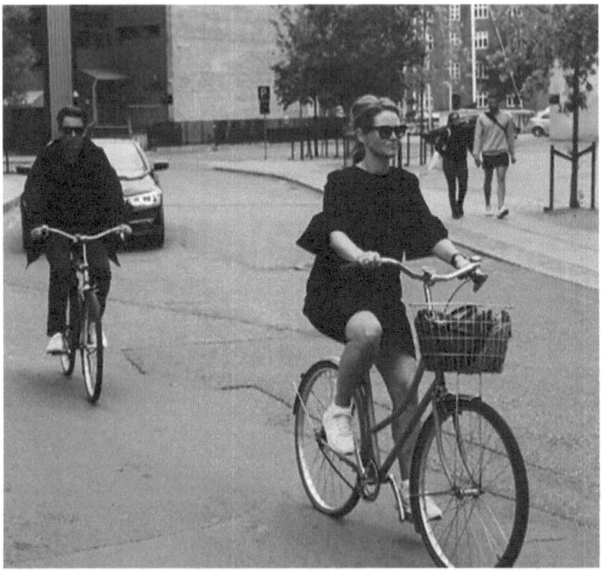

Weight is about more than appearance. Those who are overweight or obese are at a higher risk of contracting psoriasis, psoriatic arthritis, and a host of other inflammatory diseases. Obesity is a pro inflammatory state that increases the risk of high blood pressure, heart disease, and worsens autoimmune diseases. Adhering to the recommendations provided in this ebook, as well as incorporating regular exercise, will assist with weight loss and promote longer, healthier living. Additionally, maintaining a normal weight can make pharmaceuticals much more effective.

Patient story: Jim is a 50 year old stockbroker with decades long history of difficult to treat psoriasis and undiagnosed arthritis who was resistant to pharmaceutical creams and light box therapy (which is a box that mimics outdoor light). Jim was obese, had poor sleep hygiene, a high stress job, poor eating habits, and no regular exercise routine. After the first visit, he added a systemic psoriasis medication and quit his fast food habit. He was encouraged to begin a regular exercise routine that involved walking, biking, and yoga — no high intensity workouts (HIIT). After six weeks, his skin and joints were significantly less inflamed and he said he "had a new lease on life and never felt better." JA

Sleeping (It's not a Luxury, it's a necessity!)

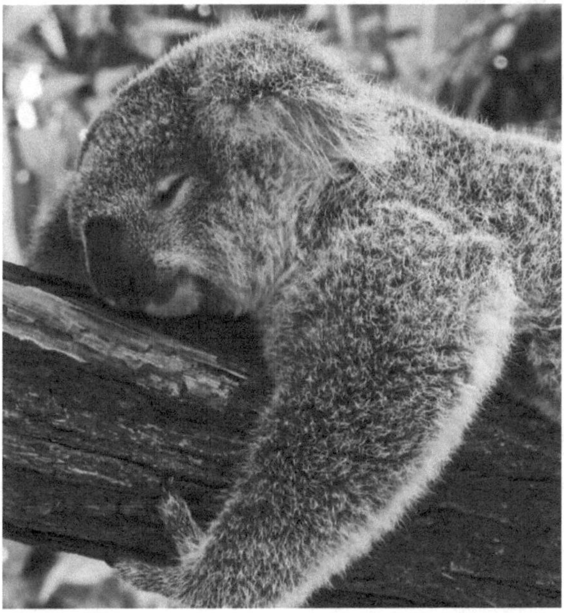

Some people wear sleep deprivation like a status symbol or a badge of honor. But science backs the benefits of getting enough sleep to allow your body and brain to recover after a day on the go. Sleep deprivation not only makes you groggy, but can increase your risk of obesity, heart disease, high blood pressure, diabetes and stroke over time. Getting 7-9 hours of rest each night is also extremely important when reducing inflammation.

Here are some suggestions to improve your sleep:

Create a consistent sleep schedule. Try to go to bed and wake up at the same time, even on weekends and vacations. This reinforces the body's inherent sleep cycle.

Create a relaxing bedtime routine, and stick with it. Take a warm shower or bath, read a book, or meditate an hour before bed.

Put away your phone or tablet an hour before bed. The blue light emitted by electronic devices decreases melatonin, and makes the brain active and alert. On Apple devices, there is a 'night mode' which, when turned on, changes the color of the screen from blue to light orange.

Consider your bedroom a sleep sanctuary. Block light with curtains, set the thermostat to 60-67 F, and get a white noise machine to block out ambient sound.

Avoid heavy late night meals, alcohol, and caffeine too close to bedtime.

How to Avoid and Eliminate Environmental Toxins

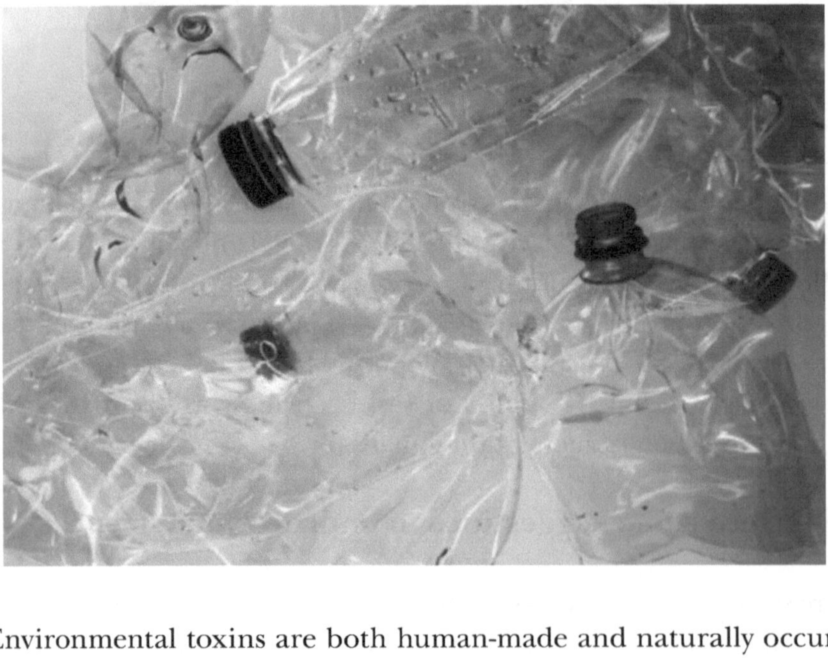

Environmental toxins are both human-made and naturally occurring substances that can harm our biological systems and health.

Some can increase the risk of cancer and act as endocrine disruptors, while others may contribute to developmental problems in children. Try to reduce exposure to toxins by filtering water with reverse osmosis, eating organic food to reduce herbicide exposure, cook with nontoxic cookware, avoid BPA exposure by reducing canned food consumption, and refraining from microwaving foods in plastic containers.

Additionally, having a bowel movement every day helps eliminate environmental toxins from the body, which may act as inflammatory triggers. Speak with your doctor if you are not having regular bowel movements every day, especially after adhering to the recommendations provided in this book.

Mind-Body Connection

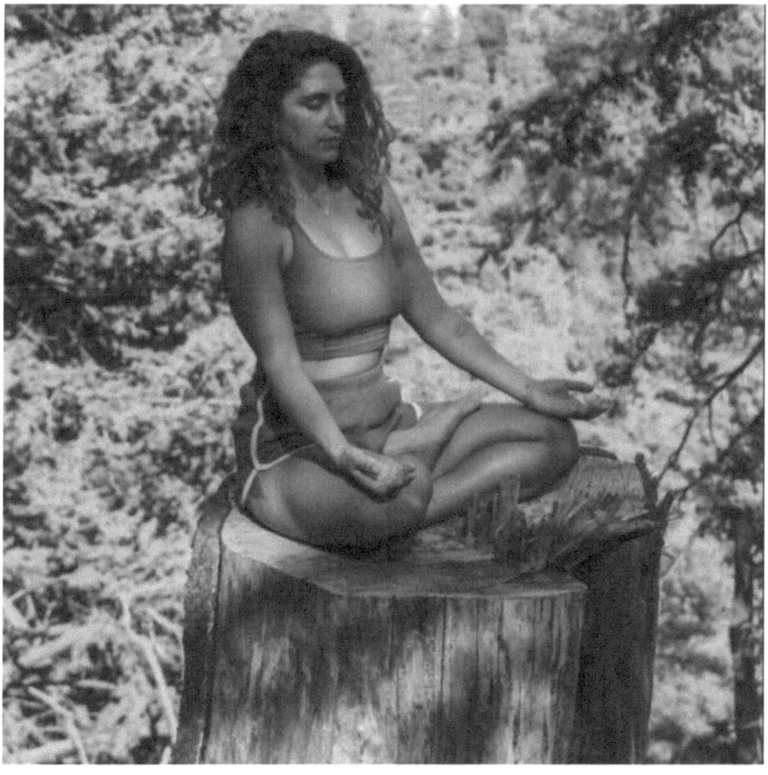

Those who are extremely stressed or suffer from depression and anxiety tend to have a higher risk of contracting psoriasis. The more stressed individuals are, the more likely they are to have poor eating and sleeping habits.

Meditating is a great way to increase happiness and reduce stress, and several apps make it easy to meditate for a few minutes each day. Try meditating for a few minutes each day with apps and websites such as Shambhala or Mindplace.

Part 3: Recipes that Can Help Control Psoriasis and Psoriatic Arthritis

BREAKFAST

Cast Iron Tofu Scramble

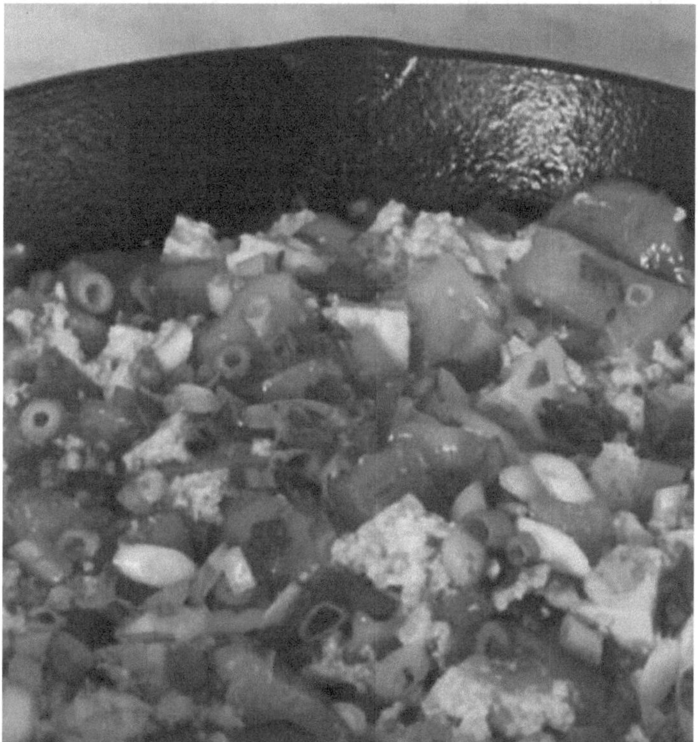

- 14 ounces of firm organic tofu, cut into ½ inch squares
- 2 bell peppers (one yellow and one green), seeded and sliced into half inch squares
- ½ cup of diced onion
- 3 tablespoons of expeller pressed grapeseed oil
- 1 teaspoon whole cumin seeds
- 1 teaspoon ground dried turmeric
- 2 tablespoons organic tamari sauce
- 1 teaspoon sesame oil
- 3 scallions, white and green parts thinly sliced for garnish
- Kosher salt

Preheat a 10 inch cast iron skillet over medium heat. Add the grapeseed oil and sauté the diced onion for 2 to 3 minutes, or until translucent. Add in the peppers and sauté for 5 to 7 minutes, or until the vegetables are soft and lightly browned. Stir in the whole cumin seeds and cook for one minute, or until the seeds are toasted and fragrant. Add the tofu to the pan along with the turmeric, tamari sauce, and sesame oil. Stir, lightly crushing the tofu squares with the back of your spoon, until combined. Continue to cook over medium heat for another five minutes until most of the liquid has evaporated and the tofu is starting to crisp.

Remove from heat, season to taste with kosher salt, and sprinkle with scallions. Serve hot with rice or millet porridge.

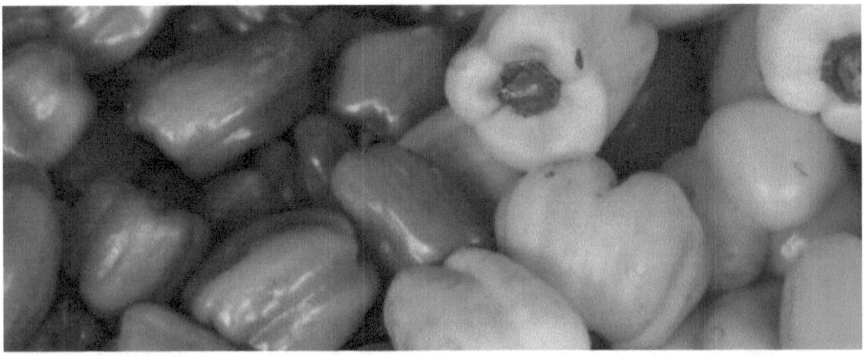

Congee-inspired Millet Instant Pot Porridge

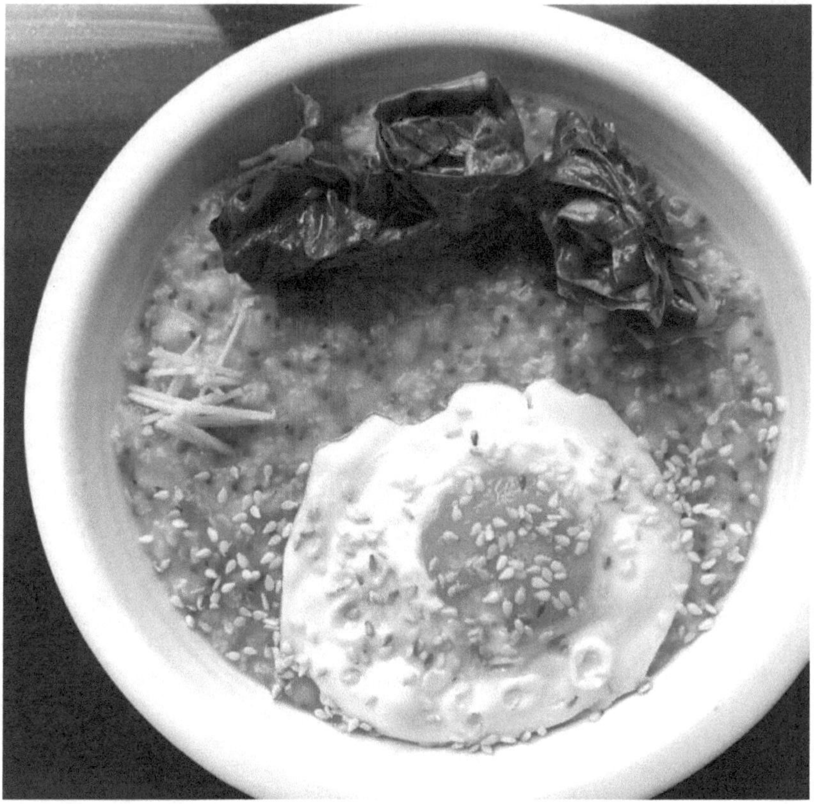

- One cup of millet
- 2 tablespoons of Chia seeds
- 2 tablespoons of hemp seeds
- 6 cups of water
- Condiments for serving: sunny side up eggs, lightly sautéed greens, slivered ginger, ground flaxseed, toasted or black sesame seeds, tamari sauce

Combine the millet, chia seeds, hemp seeds, and water in an instant pot. Fasten the lid and pressure cook for 20 minutes. You can also simply push the "porridge" button on the instant pot, and this will also cook it for 20 minutes.

After cooking, allow it to sit undisturbed for 20 to 30 minutes. Release the pressure and stir to combine. A thick porridge will be present. Ladle into bowls, and top with the condiments of your choice.

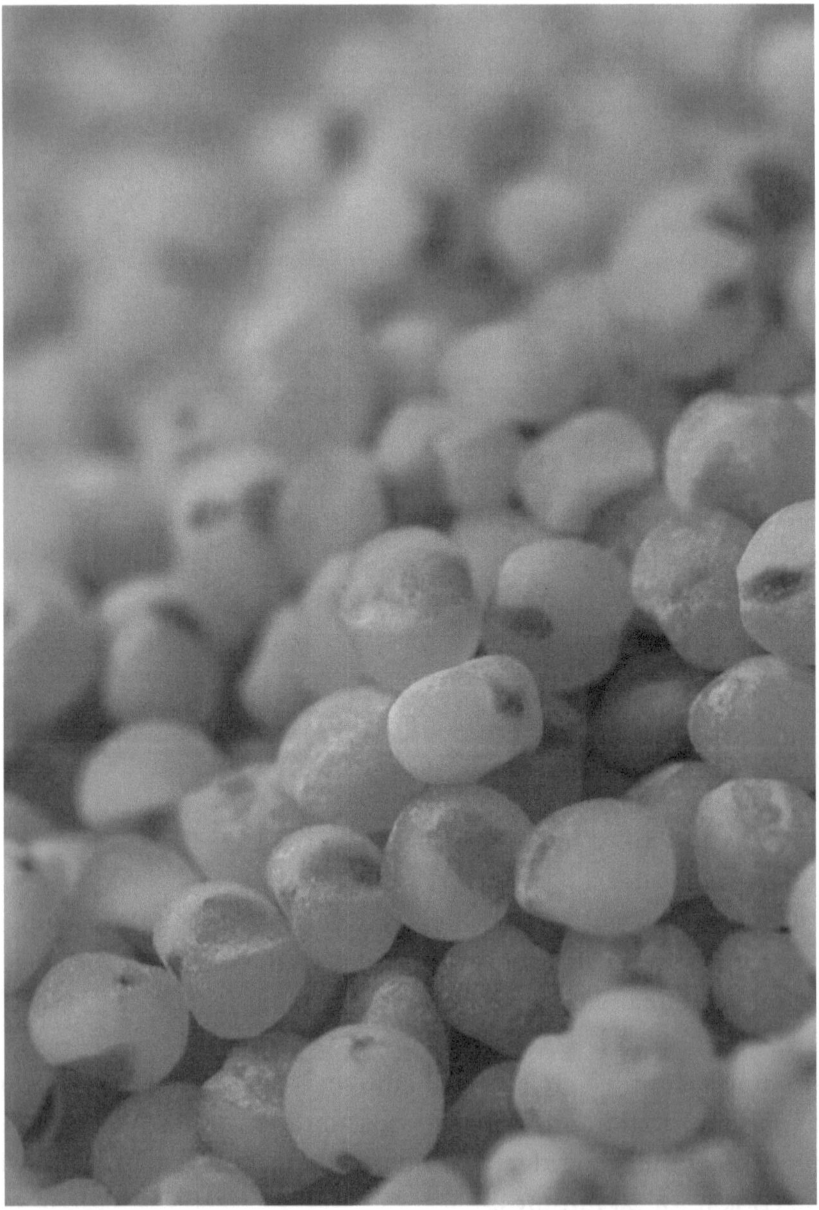

LUNCH

Basmati rice with Cumin, Peas, and Dill

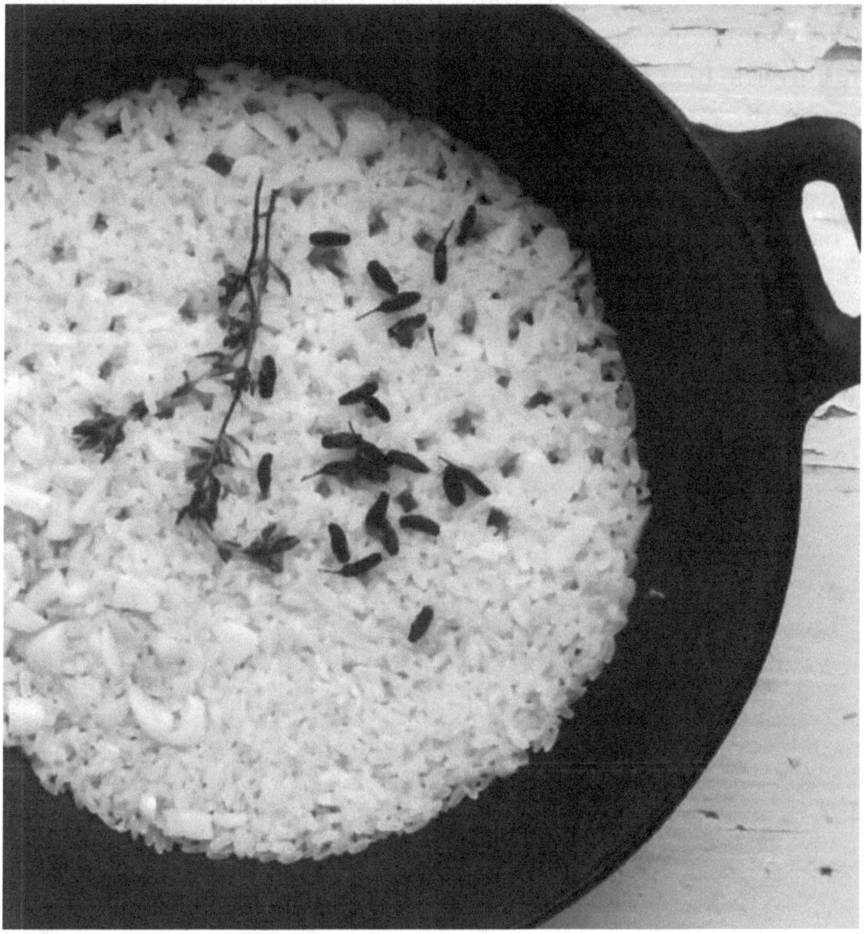

- 2 cups of basmati rice, rinsed, and soaked in water for at least 15 minutes and up to overnight, and drained
- 2 cups of frozen peas, defrosted in a cup of warm water
- 1 tablespoon of whole cumin seeds
- One cup of finely cup chopped fresh dill
- 3 tablespoons of grapeseed oil
- 2 teaspoons of kosher salt

Heat oil in a small Dutch oven with a lid until shimmering. Add the cumin seeds and toast in the oil for 1 to 2 minutes, or until fragrant. Add the drained rice and stir into the oil for 3-4 minutes, or until the rice begins to dry and toast. Add 3 cups of filtered water, 2 teaspoons of kosher salt, and bring to a boil. Cover the pan, and reduce the heat to low. Cook for 25 minutes, turn off the heat, and rest in the pan for another 10 minutes.

After the rice has rested, remove the lid. Using a fork, gently flush the rice and stir in the peas and dill. Serve hot. This makes 6-8 servings of rice and peas and will keep for a week in the refrigerator.

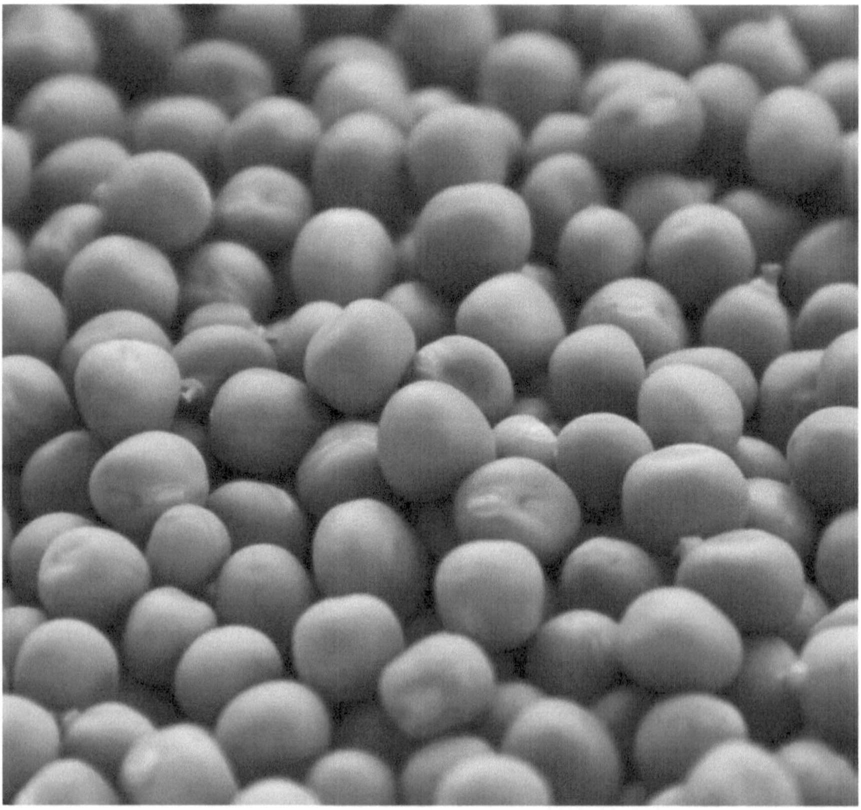

Black Lentil Burger Lettuce Wraps

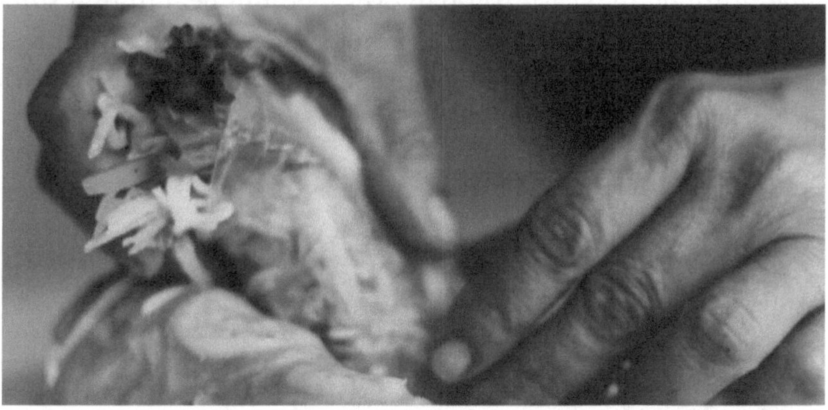

- 1 cup of black lentils
- 1 small onion, chopped
- 1 medium carrot, chopped
- ½ cup of gluten free oats
- ½ cup of walnuts
- 1 tablespoon of tamari sauce
- 2 teaspoons of sea salt
- A high heat oil such as avocado or grape seed for sautéing.
- Red leaf lettuce, organic ketchup, avocado slices, and pickles for serving

Place the black lentils in a small saucepan and cover with filtered water. Bring to a boil and then reduce to a simmer. Cook for 20 minutes, or until soft, and then drain well and set aside.

Combine the onion, carrots, oats, and walnuts in a food processor and pulse until finally chopped and a paste has formed. Add in the lentils, tamari sauce, and sea salt, and pulse again until a thick mixture forms. Scrape the mixture into a bowl. Shape half cup portions into burgers, and set the burgers onto a plate.

Refrigerate for one hour, or until firm. Heat a small amount of high temperature oil in a cast-iron pan over medium heat until it shimmers. Sauté the burgers for five minutes per side, or until nicely browned. Remove to a clean plate. Serve the burgers on lettuce with the toppings of your choice.

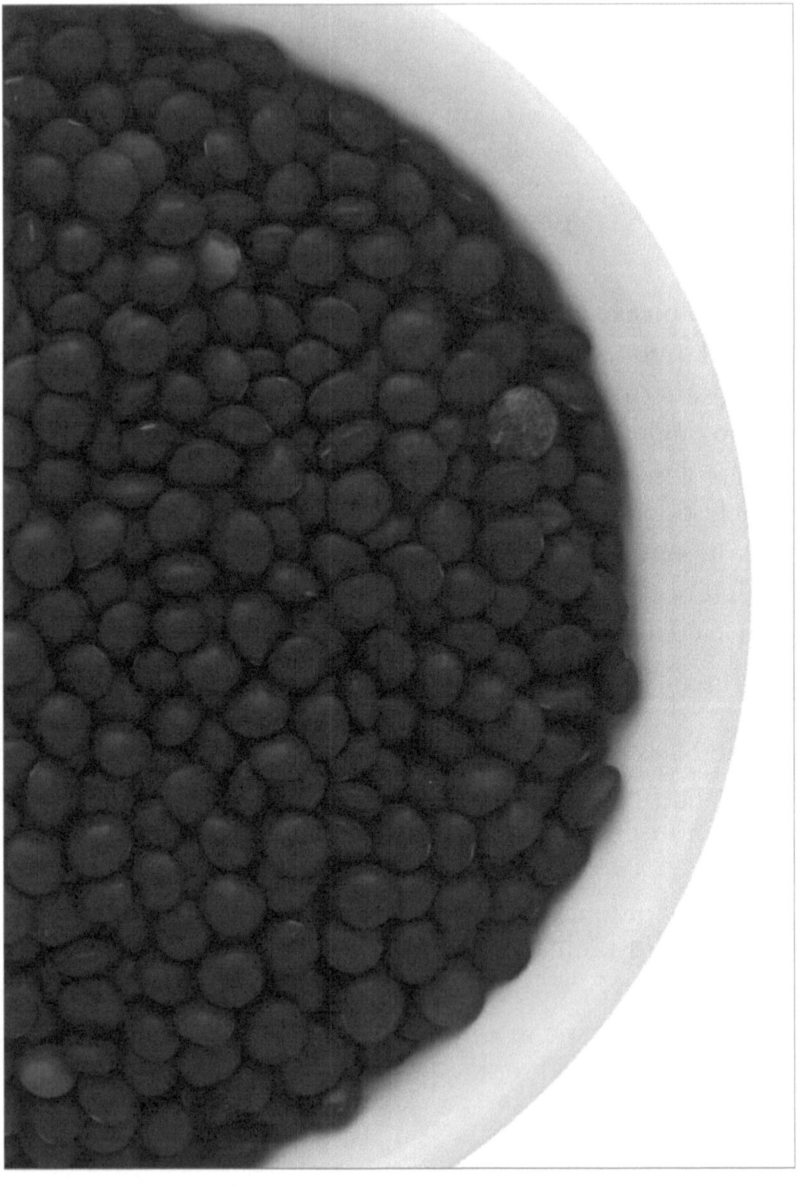

DINNER

Slow Roasted Salmon with Meyer Lemon-Caper Chutney

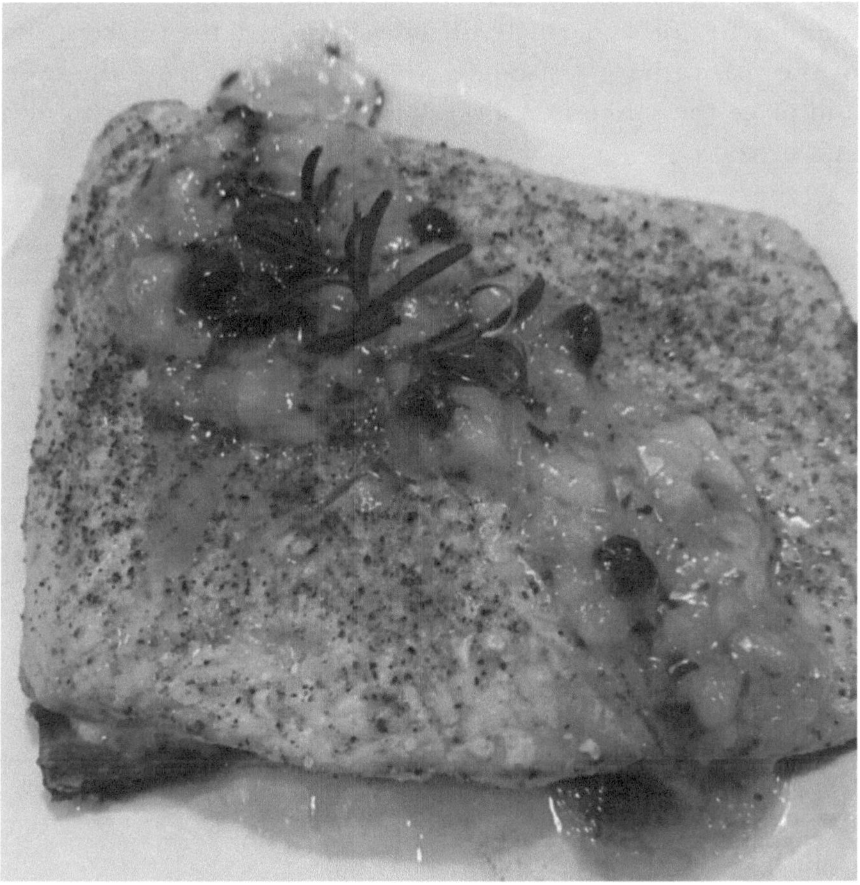

- 1 pound of center cut salmon filet; skin removed
- 1 tablespoon of olive oil
- Kosher salt and freshly ground black pepper
- One recipe of Meyer lemon-caper chutney, see below

Preheat the oven to 325 degrees. Season the salmon liberally with salt and pepper on both sides. Heat the oil over medium heat in a cast iron skillet until it shimmers. Place the salmon in the pan, skin side down. Cook over medium heat for five minutes, or until the bottom of the salmon is nicely browned.

Place the pan in the oven, and roast the salmon for 12 to 14 minutes, or until a paring knife moves through the thickest part of the fish without resistance. Remove the pan from the oven and place the salmon on a serving dish. Top with the chutney, and serve.

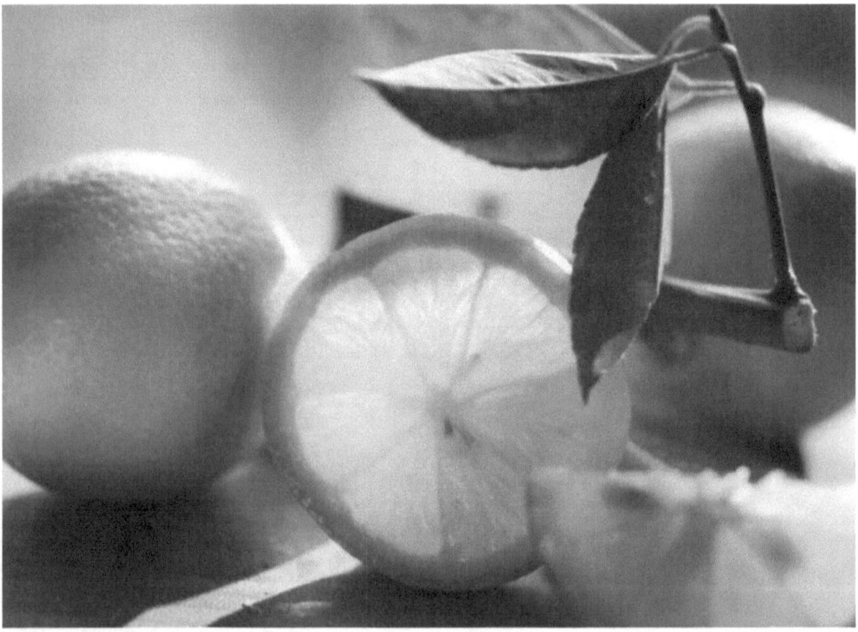

Meyer Lemon and Rosemary Compote with Capers

- Meyer lemons, washed and dried, stems and seeds removed 1/2 cup extra virgin olive oil
- teaspoon of kosher salt
- tablespoons of vinegar packed capers
- 2 teaspoons of agave syrup
- 1 tablespoon of chopped rosemary leaves

Chop the lemons and peel and flesh until minced into quarter inch pieces. Heat the olive oil in a small saucepan over medium low heat. Add the minced lemons and 1 teaspoon of kosher salt, and simmer over low heat for 30 minutes. Turn off the heat. Stir in the agave syrup, capers, and rosemary. Season to taste. Serve over the salmon.

Arctic Char with Pomegranate-Sesame Glaze over Minted Lentils

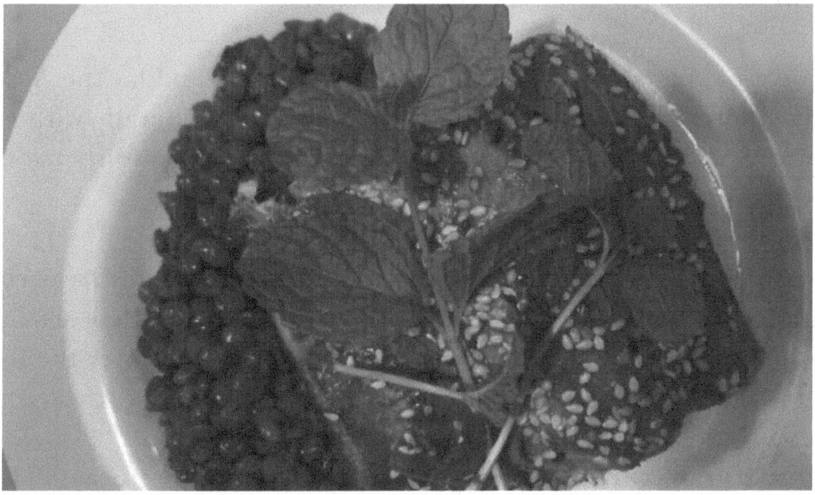

- 1 tablespoon of extra virgin olive oil
- 2 tablespoons of pomegranate molasses (this is available in many markets and online)
- 1 tablespoon of tamari sauce
- 2 teaspoons of honey
- 1 teaspoon of ground cumin seeds
- 1/2 teaspoon of ground ginger
- 1/2 teaspoon ground turmeric
- 1/2 teaspoon kosher salt
- 1 tablespoon of toasted sesame seeds
- Freshly ground pepper

- 1-1/2 pound of Arctic char filet (check www.seafoodwatch.org before buying, as the recommendations for safe fish frequently change)
- 1 recipe of minted lentils, see recipe below

Preheat the oven to 400 degrees. To make the glaze, combine the olive oil, pomegranate molasses, tamari sauce, honey, cumin, ginger, and turmeric in a small bowl, and whisk until a smooth glaze appears. Reserve 2 tablespoons of the glaze in a separate bowl.

Line a baking sheet pan with parchment paper, and lay the Arctic char filets, skin side down on the paper. Brush liberally with the glaze. Sprinkle with freshly ground pepper, and then disperse the toasted sesame seeds equally over both filets.

Roast in the oven for approximately 10 minutes, or until a paring knife passes easily through the flesh of the fish, and they are burnished nicely with glaze. Drizzle the remaining glaze over the fish. Serve hot, with the minted lentils.

How to cook minted lentils:

- 1 cup of organic brown or French Puy lentils
- 1 teaspoon of kosher salt
- 2 tablespoons of extra virgin olive oil
- 1 teaspoon whole cumin seeds
- 3 tablespoons of thinly sliced fresh mint leaves

Bring a small saucepan of water to boil, and add the lentils. Lower the heat to a simmer, and cook for 25 to 30 minutes, or until soft. Turn off the flame, and mix in one teaspoon of kosher salt to the water and lentil mixture. Leave for three minutes, and then taste the lentils for seasoning. If they require more seasoning, leave them for another two minutes in the salted water and then taste again.

Once the lentils are properly seasoned, drain them into a strainer. Wipe the saucepan clean. Return the saucepan to the stove, add the olive oil and cumin seeds, and heat until the cumin seeds are fragrant, one to two minutes. Add the lentils and mint leaves, and stir to combine. Taste for seasoning, and serve with the fish.

Fried Forbidden Rice with Tofu and Kimchi

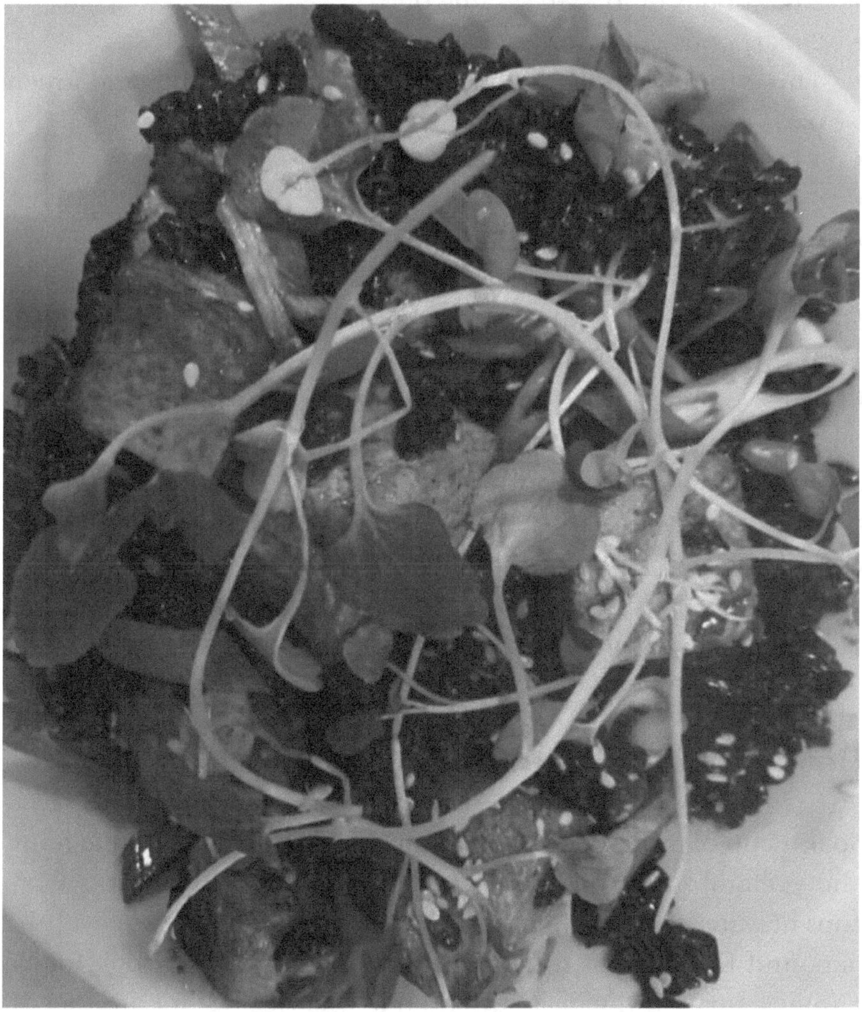

Three cups of cooked forbidden (black) rice, see directions below

- 14 ounces of organic, firm tofu, cut into half inch cubes
- 1/2 cup of cabbage kimchi, julienned into fine strips
- 3 tablespoons of expeller pressed grape seed oil or expeller pressed avocado oil
- 2 tablespoons of organic tamari sauce
- 2 teaspoons of toasted sesame oil
- 2 teaspoons of agave syrup
- Three thinly sliced scallions, include both the white and green parts
- 1 tablespoon of toasted sesame seeds
- Several handfuls of baby watercress
- Gojuchang paste to taste

Heat the grape seed oil in a large frying pan over medium heat, until it shimmers. Add the tofu squares, and sauté until lightly browned on both sides. Add in the rice and kimchi, and mix thoroughly with the tofu. Combine the tamari sauce, sesame oil, and agave in a measuring cup, and stir into the rice mixture. Continue to cook over medium-high heat until the rice crisps on the bottom of the pan, about 5 minutes, stirring occasionally. Turn off the heat. Sprinkle with the sliced scallions and sesame seeds, and mound the baby watercress on top. Serve hot with gojuchang paste on the side.

How to cook forbidden rice:

Soak 1 cup of forbidden rice in plenty of water for at least one hour, and preferably overnight. Discard the soaking water. Bring 1-1/2 cups of water to a boil in a small saucepan. Add the rice, cover the pan, and bring down the flame to its lowest setting. Cook for 25 minutes, turn off the heat, and then let the rice rest for another 10 minutes.

Sautéed Kale with Crispy Mushrooms

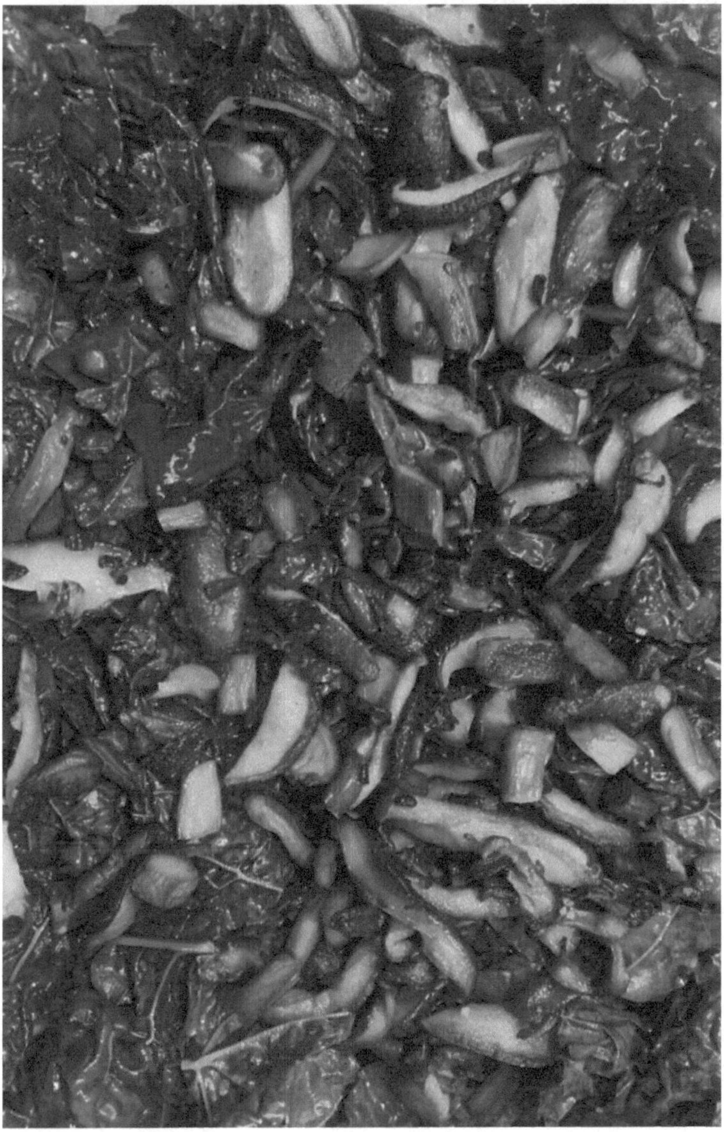

- 12 ounces of organic shiitake mushrooms, stems removed, and caps sliced into quarter inch strips
- Two handfuls of Tuscan kale, woody stems removed, and leaves sliced into 2-inch pieces

- Two garlic cloves, thinly sliced
- 4 tablespoons of olive oil
- One tablespoon of apple cider vinegar
- Kosher salt and freshly ground black pepper

Heat 2 tablespoons of olive oil in a large saucepan over medium heat. Add mushrooms and sauté, stirring frequently, until browned and crispy, about seven or eight minutes. Season lightly with kosher salt and black pepper, and remove the mushrooms to a plate. Add two more tablespoons of olive oil to the pan. Add the garlic and cook over medium heat for 1 to 2 minutes, or until golden and fragrant. Then add the sliced kale to the pan. Using tongs, turn the kale gently into the garlic and oil until wilted. This will take 2 to 3 minutes. Stir in the apple cider vinegar. Turn off the heat, add the mushrooms back into the pan, and stir to combine. Season again lightly with salt and pepper. This makes 6 to 8 servings of sautéed greens, and will keep for a week.

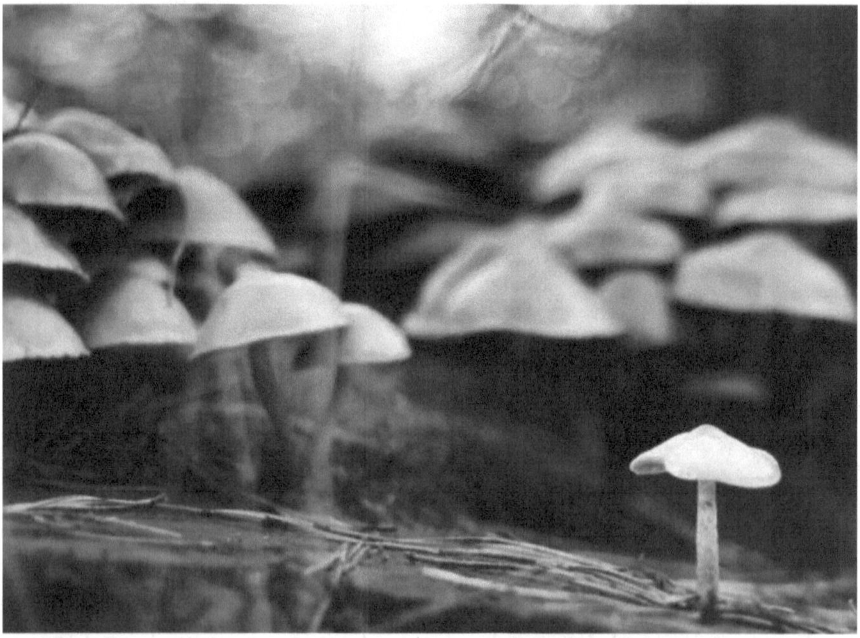

DESSERT

Berry Compote

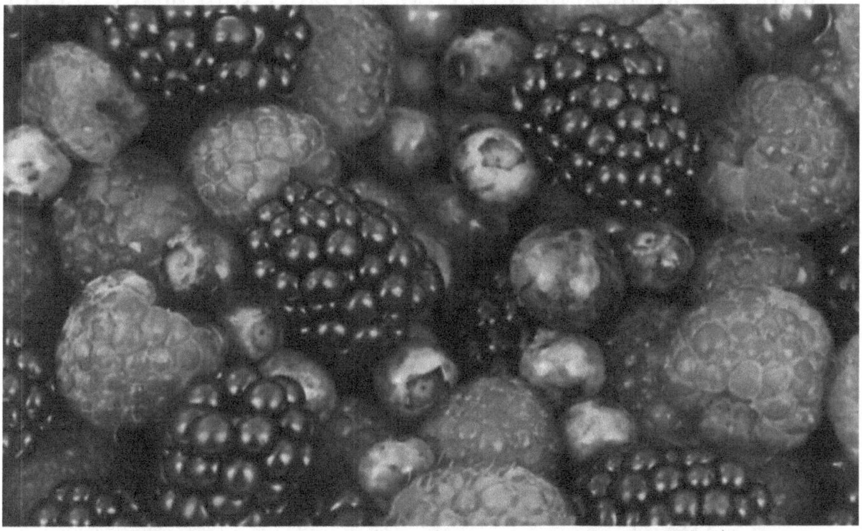

- 3.5 cups of frozen organic blackberries, raspberries, and blueberries
- One cinnamon stick, broken in half, or ½ teaspoon of ground cinnamon
- 1 to 2 tablespoons of honey Combine the frozen berries and cinnamon in a large saucepan. Cook over low heat, stirring occasionally, until the berries have melted and a thick sauce has formed. Turn off the heat. Stir in the honey, 1 tablespoon at a time, or until sweet to taste. Allow to cool, and store in a glass jar.

Serve in small glasses on its own, over yogurt, or sprinkled with granola and ground flaxseed.

"Let food be thy medicine, thy medicine shall be thy food."
– Hippocrates

"The fork is your most powerful tool to change your health and the planet. Food is the most powerful medicine to heal chronic illness."
– Dr Mark Hyman

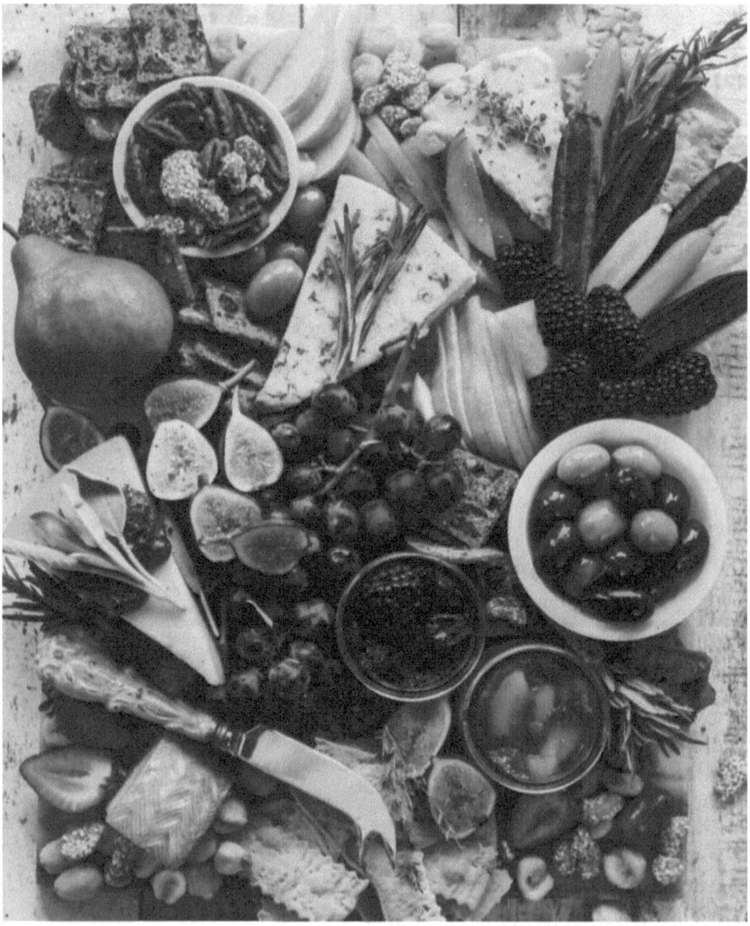

Made in United States
Troutdale, OR
10/18/2026

56022114R00037